THE HEALING POWER OF COMPASSION

Compassion
arises through ceaseless
manifestations, as the stories
collected in this book demonstrate.
Through their lucid and memorable insights,
these stories lead us to one fundamental truth:
Compassion is the essence of all authentic
spirituality and transcends any definitions
and differences of religions.

His Eminence Chagdud Tulku Rinpoche,
author, *Lord of the Dance* and
Gates to Buddhist Practice

THE HEALING POWER OF COMPASSION

The Essence of Buddhist Acts

Compiled and Edited by
PAMELA BLOOM

Foreword by
JOAN HALIFAX ROSHI

New Age Books

ISBN: 81-7822-227-2

First Indian Edition: Delhi, 2006

(Earlier published 2000 by Conari Press, USA)

Published by
NEW AGE BOOKS
A-44 Naraina Phase-I
New Delhi-110 028 (INDIA)
Email: nab@vsnl.in
Website: www.newagebooksindia.com

For Sale in Indian Subcontinent Only

Printed in India
at Shri Jainendra Press
A-45 Naraina Phase-I, New Delhi-110 028

To my parents,

who transmitted to me

the genes of compassion,

and to my teachers,

who nourish them

By the power and truth of these teachings
May all beings enjoy happiness and the causes
of happiness
Be free from sorrow and the causes of sorrow.
May they never be separated from the sacred
happiness that is sorrowless
And may they all live, safely and in freedom
believing in the equality of all that lives.

CONTENTS

FOREWORD

by Joan Halifax Roshi,

author of *A Buddhist Life in America* and *Being with Dying*

Sharing stories is as old as fire.

Through the sharing of dreams, visions, and rites of passages, tribal societies discovered who they were, where they came from, and where they were going. Through stories they learned how to love, how to fight, how to reconcile, and how to live and dance with the unmediated elements.

Today, when we share stories about the deepest moments of our lives, we also bear witness to what makes our crazed, myopic, twenty-four nonstop hours more meaningful, transcendent, and most of all, healing. In sharing our stories we bear witness to both our differences and our union.

In my work with the dying, as I've sat at the bedsides of people with catastrophic illnesses, I've noticed one story being told over and over again. Fully facing the truth of one's own impermanence can open up a flood of tenderness and compassion that often heals the deepest wounds. I think of Patrick, who had Kaposi's sarcoma and who wanted to live longer just so he could take on the suffering of all men with KS. Or Lily, who was able to let go of a lifetime of resentment and receive the love of her daughter, just hours before her passing. But we don't have to wait until we are deathly ill to open our hearts. The practice of meditation, as taught by the Buddha, gives us that same opportunity to discover who we are—by waking us up to our greatest vulnerability and our greatest potential. And, as Bernie Glassman, my friend and dharma brother, says in this book, "The function of that awakening is learning how to serve."

The wonderful stories that Pamela Bloom has collected give us a precious glimpse into the heart of service the Buddha discovered more than 2,600 years ago. Poignant and courageous, these modern stories show that Buddhism is not a dry, dusty religion but a vibrant, engaged path with practical solutions for today's real problems. Whether exalted lamas or ordinary students, the practitioners in this book have taken daring leaps into the unknown of their own being—into what might be called "visionary compassion." That is to say, compassion that goes the extra mile beyond one's comfort level, compassion that embraces self and other as one continuum, compassion that sees the world squarely for what it is, yet neither flinches nor gives up. It is a state of mind, a condition of being, that we all desperately need.

In this new millennium we have the opportunity to create something wonderful or something disastrous with our lives, with each other, and with the planet. Even the scientists today tell us our global survival depends not only our brains but on our hearts. But it will also take guts. May the stories that we choose to weave at this linchpin of time help to empower our hearts, embolden our brains, and lead us all—together—to higher and deeper ground.

EVERY BREATH WE TAKE

My religion is kindness.

—His Holiness the Dalai Lama

There is, strictly speaking, no such thing as a Buddhist act of compassion. A genuine Buddhist practitioner would never be interested in labeling any act *Buddhist,* let alone one of compassion. In the Buddhist teachings, compassion is universal. Even Mother Theresa has said, "Religion has nothing to do with compassion."

And yet there is a very special flavor that the Buddhist teachings can bring to the understanding and experience of compassion, no matter what one's religious affiliation may be. It is said that the Buddha Shakyamuni himself did not suddenly achieve enlightenment from the efforts of one lifetime; rather it was the merit accumulated from a thousand lifetimes of selfless acts that created the ground for his ultimate enlightenment. By the time he lived as a prince, and even though his father desperately wanted to shield him from the harsher realities of life, Prince

Siddhartha held deep within his mindstream the desire, the passion, to achieve enlightenment for the sake of others. Indeed, his ultimate experience of enlightenment only further clarified that compassion is inseparable from the view that all life is both impermanent and yet inextricably interrelated, and that the root of all suffering is to imagine it otherwise.

Why does anyone pursue the truth of the Buddha? It was the search to understand my own personal suffering that led me to the study of meditation and the Buddhist teachings. In 1978, following the loss of my singing voice in music school, I was thrown into a deep depression and began a spiritual quest, intuitively sensing that the search for my voice and the search for the divine were the same. One weekend I found myself deep in the hill country of Texas at a meditation retreat led by Ösel Tendzin, the senior-most student of Chögyam Trungpa Rinpoche, the Tibetan master responsible for first bringing the teachings of Tibetan Buddhism to the West. All weekend I either fell asleep or fidgeted painfully, but whenever Ösel Tendzin spoke, I sat on the edge of my cushion; here was a spark like none I had ever seen. In a private interview, as we sat perched on two chairs alone in the middle of a vast meadow, he told me how to heal my voice and my spirit.

"Develop 360-degree vision," he said.

It sounded impressive, but I didn't have a clue what he was talking about until several years later when, as a music critic, I interviewed the great jazz vocalist Bobby McFerrin. A daring improviser, McFerrin is known for using his voice in both playful and profound ways, in techniques drawn from deep meditative states. When I asked why it seemed that his performances were all marked by an extraordinary compassion, he told me, "I don't know why, but sometimes at the end of a concert, there's no me, no performer left, there's only an audience."

Strange as it may seem, there was something in that statement that helped me begin to understand the nature of the Buddha's compassion. More than anything, compassion as taught by the Buddha is not about a giver and receiver, an "I" and an other. In fact, the various Buddhist meditation practices taught to develop compassion are all focused on the dissolution of the abyss between that which gives and that which receives—that is to say, the dissolution of the *perception* of that abyss. No me, no you, only a sea of sentient beings suffering for endless eons, all looking for a way out. The Buddha says the "way out," the cure and the antidote, the medicine and the balm, lies deep within us, in the very nature of who we are.

In order to understand the nature of that suffering and the nature of liberation, the Buddha's teachings have traditionally begun with looking into oneself, into the roots of one's own anger, resentment, passion, jealousy, ignorance, and greed. At the core of human misery, the Buddha said, is our self-centeredness, our clinging to a solid frozen self that we imagine to be permanent. The practice of meditation helps awaken our awareness to this fundamental habit of clinging and allows the possibility of cutting through it. Slowly, by coming to know one's own habits of mind intimately, we can choose to be no longer imprisoned by them, and we can actually begin to work with other sentient beings *as they are,* without the obstacle of our own neurotic projections.

As we slowly peel away the layers of our projections and "undress" our minds, what arises in our experience, the teachings say, is something so vast, so vibrant, so healing and miraculous, so beyond concept, as to be accessible only though *direct* experience. For most of us, even after years of meditating, such an experience comes first only in the merest of glimpses, no longer than the blink of an eye and just as ephemeral. For fully realized masters, however, the state is all-pervasive, beyond time and space, and able to be transmitted to others who are open to it. There are no words to describe this state, except un-words, for it is the very lack of mental labeling that defines it. But what is truly extraordinary, the Buddha says, is that this state, though beyond construct, is not static but rather full of "life," the ultimate union of wisdom and compassion. In fact, this state *is* us and has always been us. It is our birthright and our very being's inheritance, merely obscured by our mental clouds of passion, aggression, and ignorance.

With the awakening to this quality of mind, which is called in Sanskrit *bodhichitta,** compassionate action takes on unlimited dimension. Loving sentiment begins to arise out of our deepest connection to all life, not from a concept or romantic illusion. Action become appropriate to the situation, without leaving any messy imprint of the "do-gooder." Generosity becomes unlimited, yet there is no danger of martyrdom or self-sacrifice for

* The calligraphy of the Sanskrit word "bodhichitta" or "awakened heart" on page 13 was made expressly for this book by the Tibetan master Sogyal Rinpoche before his public talk on April 16, 2000, at the Synod House of St. John the Divine Cathedral, New York City, in front of about fifteen devoted members of the Rigpa sangha. Calligraphies by such masters are said to transmit the very energy of the word itself.

there is simply nothing to lose. Energy needed to accomplish a task becomes no different than the motivation that propels it. There are many stories of the Buddha throughout countless lifetimes giving himself body and soul to the benefit of another—for example, the time he offered his flesh and blood to a hungry tigress who needed food for her cub. But in viewing this story from the point of view of bodhichitta, we can see that the Buddha was only acting as naturally as he could, the *only* way he could, in total and undilutable joy.

Such selflessness, however, seems almost unattainable by normal standards, or is it? Once, in a snug, comfortable loft in New York's Soho district, I remember hearing a teaching by Kyabje Gelek Rinpoche, a vibrant Tibetan master, in which he asked what would we do if someone armed with a gun stormed in and threatened to kill us all. Most of us agreed we would probably duck under a chair at the first hint of threat. But how many of us, he asked, would actually throw ourselves in front of the gun in order to protect another? The dilemma he proposed to us seemed vaguely hypothetical until three weeks later, at Columbine High School in Littleton, Colorado, when a math teacher lost his life throwing himself in front of his students in order to protect them from two gun-wielding classmates. Dave

Sanders wasn't a Buddhist, as far as I know, but nothing could more symbolize the selfless courage of the Buddha's compassion than that singular act. Truly he deserves to be called what is known in the Buddhist tradition as a great Bodhisattva, one who has totally and uncompromisingly dedicated his life to saving other sentient beings. One can only imagine how deep the wish, the prayer, to be of benefit to others, must have been implanted in his heart, to have acted so swiftly, so surely, without thought. The potential to be a Bodhisattva, says the Buddha, is inside all of us.

For most people, however, the development of compassion must necessarily start small, and the various Buddhist traditions have a richness of methods to cultivate loving-kindness even in the most intransigent of beings. In the Tibetan tradition, there is a practice called *Tonglen,* a meditation in which you mentally inhale the suffering of other beings in the form of dark clouds or smoke, and exhale love and compassion in the form of light. In Theravadin Buddhism there is a practice called *Metta,* or loving-kindness, in which you extend the wish to all beings that they may be happy, well, and free from suffering.

These are emotional-spiritual exercises of the mind that must be done over and over again, especially for one's enemies, but they are powerful, for they reach far into the dark recesses of one's heart, into the very resistance of that self that clings to one's own happiness at the expense of others. In the back of this book, you will find short versions of these practices, and I urge you to try them. In a sense, they are a form of active prayer, for the more you do them, the more you will feel their effects, and the more you will cultivate not only a deeper understanding of yourself, but also the wisdom, empathy, generosity, equanimity, and patience to work with others. In essence you will lose yourself and gain the world.

More than anything, this book is about the living Buddha in all of us, and many stories shared here show the power of these practices in ways both marvelous and miraculous; I assure you they are true. In visiting patients as a hospital chaplain, in working with those suffering from catastrophic illnesses, in dealing with the everyday relationship problems of my own life, I have found these practices to be indispensable, not only in keeping my own sanity but also in developing into the kind of person who at the very least aspires to relieve the suffering of others, not cause them further grief.

Not all of us, however, are interested in standing up to snipers or running off to Bosnia to negotiate cease-fires. But even the smallest act of compassion can have enormous effect. The latest environmental theories in vogue these days recognize that even the tiniest flutter of a butterfly's wings can affect life on the other side of the planet. This book, full of stories drawn from both masters and students in many traditions of Buddhism, including Zen, Tibetan, Chinese, Vietnamese, Cambodian, and nondenominational, is meant to inspire by the examples of those who have taken the Buddhist teachings to heart and struggled to apply them to their daily lives. You will find stories about compassion in the workplace, on the city streets of New York, behind prison walls, in the middle of war. You will find stories about the power of meditation to transform the so-called justified anger of social protest into a shared well of understanding. You will find stories about the magical power of prayer—to heal wounds, stop bullets, to change the flow of the elements. Simply, these stories show that when the mind and heart unite in the view that the separate self we imagine ourselves to be is an illusion, anything is possible. And it is possible *today,* not just in the Buddha's time.

The Buddhist teachings are vast, and the greatest merit a book like this can achieve is to inspire you to delve more deeply into the traditional teachings. If the words and stories of the dedicated practitioners in this book touch your heart, I encourage you to seek out a living teacher who can bring to full life the thoughts, words, and actions of the Buddha himself. To meet an enlightened master is to be afforded the opportunity to take part in a living transmission of wisdom and compassion that has been in effect ever since Shakyamuni himself achieved enlightenment—a breathing, vibrant lineage of those dedicated without the slightest hesitation to work for the benefit of others. For Tibetans, and now for many around the world, His Holiness the Dalai Lama is the epitome of the greatest Bodhisattva, and there are numerous stories in this book about personal contact with him that has changed the course of lives forever. Surely, there is nothing more contagious than pure compassion, but its power is often mysterious and one never knows exactly when seeds planted long ago in a moment of rare openness will suddenly sprout.

In 1983, while on a three-month retreat in Pennsylvania, I decided, after much consideration, to take the traditional Bodhisattva vow in ceremony with Chögyam Trungpa Rinpoche. As was Rinpoche's habit in those days, the student would enter his study for a minute, wait nervously for his attention until he finally looked up, flashed on your essence, then retreated privately to write in beautiful calligraphy the name he had chosen for you. When I finally received my name, Compassion Dharma Lake, I was hugely disappointed. A lake did not sound so big and certainly not as glamorous and fierce as the name my friend received, something having to do with a tigress. But traditionally a Bodhisattva name is one you must earn, one that shows the qualities you must struggle with and develop in your lifetime with regard to other people. How did Trungpa Rinpoche know that even though I come from a family deeply devoted to service, I myself would spend the next seventeen years of my life in a constant struggle to learn how to apply compassion to every aspect of my life? So it is my deepest prayer that this book, filled with the compassionate hearts of so many, become a lake of compassion for each reader, one in which you may ultimately realize something of the Buddha's teaching and catch a glimpse, a reflection, of your own true nature. If this book sparks even the slightest awareness that life on this planet could be something other than a morass of conflict, violence, and despair, its efforts will have been well worth it. For those seeking to relieve suffering and develop the ultimate source of healing within, may this book be a boat, a bridge, a passage.

Pamela Bloom

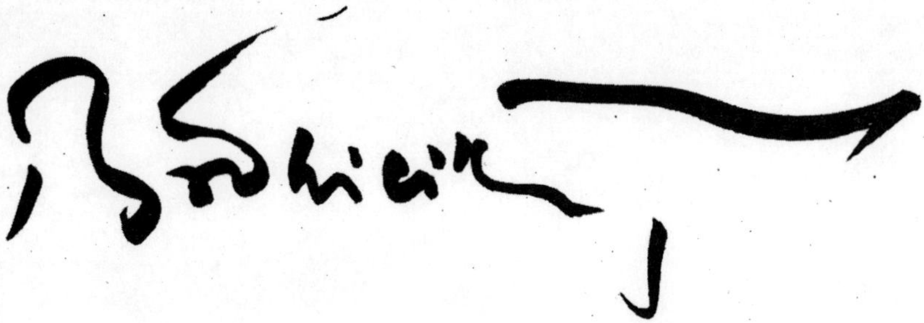

A beautiful word or thought that is not
accompanied by corresponding acts is
like a bright flower that bears no fruit.
It would not produce any effect.

The Buddha

The Stories

FROM VICTIM TO LIBERATOR

I was on a meditation retreat in the south of France when a visiting master was introduced to the group. An audience of over three hundred Western students of Buddhism waited quietly for him to speak. He was about forty years old, quite tall and broad-shouldered for a Tibetan, with an enormous presence like a mountain, though he barely smiled. As he began to talk he repeatedly wiped at his draining right eye, as if something in him was constantly crying, but his voice remained strong. Soon his personal story unfolded.

For fifteen years, as a young man, this Rinpoche and his elderly master had been imprisoned inside Tibet as victims of Chinese persecution. Although he did not go into details, the conditions they had had to endure were of the roughest sort, with many days spent chained together in their dark, dirty cell. The Chinese, he said, not content with normal torture, had been determined to persecute devout Tibetans in the worst possible way by denying them the right to meditate; every time their eyes closed they were beaten. But because the Chinese did not understand that Tibetans actually meditate with their eyes open, the two were able to continue their prayers and meditations in secret. Unfortunately, as the years went by, the abuse only got worse; in fact, Rinpoche's constantly tearing eye was the result of beatings from that time. He had even had to endure the loss of his master, who died next to him one night in their cell. After many years of torture, escape from this living hell had come to seem impossible.

But then one day, out of the blue, two of the jailers addressed him directly: "What are you doing?" they said. "No matter what we do to you, now matter how we hurt you, nothing moves you." Apparently the jailers had practiced all sorts of martial arts, but they had finally met a power they didn't understand. "You know something we don't," they told him, "and because we are the jailers, we must learn it in order to become stronger than you."

So because he had no other weapon, he taught his jailers the very practice he and his master had been doing—the Tibetan meditation called Tonglen, which is the practice of breathing in the suffering of others and breathing out light. It was the same practice that many of us had been learning at this retreat with some struggle, for to actually take on the suffering of others with no sense of martyrdom or resentment is a great affront to one's ego. So, to imagine that this monk and his elderly master had found the inspiration to not only practice compassion but to teach it in the middle of hell to the very beings who were the agents of their suffering . . . well, that was a level of compassion that transcends the ordinary mind.

And yet, that is the essence of Buddhist compassion. And as a result, as Rinpoche told it, the unbelievable happened.

One day, some time later, the Chinese jailers suddenly announced to their Tibetan captive that they were releasing him from jail. No reason. Just his time was up. And they set him free.

And that is how he came to be before us on that bright sunny day in the south of France, with his eye running like a persistent rain of remembrance, his gaze brilliantly clear, his posture immovable like a warrior's. In fact, as I remember it now, there was not even a trace of resentment in his voice, only perhaps the bittersweet irony that his master had not lived to see that somewhere between the in-breath and the out-breath, the boundary between persecutor and persecuted had finally dissolved.

—*Pamela Bloom*

An effortless compassion can arise for all beings who have not realized their true nature. So limitless is it that if tears could express it, you would cry without end.

—*Nyoshul Khenpo Rinpoche*

TAKING ON THE SUFFERING OF OTHERS

In a previous life, the Buddha was born in a hell where the inhabitants were forced to pull wagons. He was harnessed to a wagon with another person called Kamarupa, but the two of them were too weak to get their vehicle to move. The guards goaded them on and beat them with red-hot weapons, causing them incredible suffering.

The future Buddha thought, "Even with two of us together we can't get the wagon to move, and each of us is suffering as much as the other. I'll pull it and suffer alone, so that Kamarupa can be relieved."

He said to the guards, "Put his harness over my shoulders. I'm going to pull the cart on my own."

But the guards just got angry. "Who can do anything to prevent others from experiencing the effects of their own actions?" they said and beat him about the head with their clubs.

Because of this good thought, however, the Buddha immediately left that life in hell and was reborn in a celestial realm. It is said that this was how he first began to benefit others.

—*Patrul Rinpoche, from* The Words of My Perfect Teacher

THE HIGHEST PRAYER

Some of the first dharma students in the West like John Giorno, Allen Ginsburg, and William Burroughs had invited Dudjom Rinpoche [one of the most extraordinary Tibetan meditation masters of the last century] to come to the United States, and I had the great honor to travel with him as his translator on his first Atlantic flight. I remember I was sitting next to him in the plane when we flew over, and there was one moment when he looked through the window and said softly, "All those I fly over, may they all be liberated." He said it in a particular way, so quietly and unobtrusively: he was not boasting, he was not saying that he had the power to do this, but just in the humblest way imaginable, ". . . may all these beings be liberated." And I thought, "How extraordinary: this master really does have that power." But it was because of his prayers as well. It did not mean they were all going to be liberated. Rather, through the power of his prayer, he would have become the *cause* of their liberation. *That* is bodhichitta.

—*Sogyal Rinpoche, in a public talk*

> Could we exclude any from our compassion any more than the sun could exclude any from the warmth and radiance of its rays?
>
> — *Chagdud Tulku Rinpoche*

HEART SURGERY

I was in a great deal of pain growing up as a teenager in Brazil. Although I had a very good life in the worldly sense, I was very frustrated and didn't understand why. In fact, I was smoking pain and anger and making everyone around me miserable too. Wanting to help, some friends invited me to see a teacher known for her healing abilities. I was very skeptical that any spiritual teacher would be able to help me. I believe that she perceived my skepticism immediately upon our meeting because she was very fierce and strong with me. She literally threw a coin at my face and when it hit the floor she said, "See this coin? It has two sides. One side is your spiritual life and you must take care of it. The other is your worldly life and with that only suffering will remain in you." After those few words, she proceeded to kick me out of her house. I was shocked by her words and left with an anger that would stay with me for months.

One year later, still frustrated and distressed, my life had become unbearable. There was a terrible pain in my heart and I felt practically suicidal. One day, as I was driving to work in terrible despair, suddenly the image of this woman throwing the coin at me came into my mind. So I decided to try to find her. I started driving wildly around Rio de Janeiro, a big city that is difficult to get around, looking for her home. My friends had taken me there the first time so I didn't know exactly where she lived, but my motivation and will were so strong that I would not give up. After hours and hours of driving up and down the city streets, I became so desperate that I leaned my head on the steering wheel and broke into tears. Suddenly I felt someone tapping on my shoulder. A woman, a stranger, started telling me that I ought to talk to someone and suggested I go to this address she gave me. I didn't think much of it, but because I was so desperate I decided to go. When I made the final turn and looked up, I was astonished to see the woman I had met one year before standing in front of her modest home. A seventy-eight-year old woman, she was very sick and very weak, but she had one incredible smile and a powerful will. She came over to me and said, "Oh, son, it took so long for you to flip the coin over. I am so happy you came." She was so warm and so nurturing that I spent the day crying in her arms. She didn't say much, just a few words, but they would prove to be the words of my first spiritual teacher: "It's all right, son, now you are on the path."

I studied healing with this teacher until her death many years later. She created all the conditions for me to embrace my spiritual path, until I found my ultimate path in Tibetan Buddhism. Today, inspired by my goal to spread the buddhadharma, I shoulder many responsibilities as a teacher and director of two monasteries and many dharma centers. But I know I am who I am today because of the kindness of this first great teacher who tossed a coin in my face and threw me out of her house. That's what I cultivate and remember in the midst of my greatest difficulties—how in one moment of great compassion she so skillfully and invisibly opened my heart.

—Venerable Segyu Choepel Rinpoche

I'm not a therapist. I don't know how to therapute people. But I know one thing: anger is very expensive.

—Kyabje Gelek Rinpoche

TWO MINDS, ONE HEART

About fifteen years ago, I used to help a committee for orphans, victims of the war in Vietnam. From Vietnam, they sent out applications, one sheet of paper with a small picture of a child in the corner, telling the name, the age, and the condition of the orphan. We were supposed to translate it from Vietnamese into French, English, Dutch, or German in order to seek a sponsor, so that the child would have food to eat and books for school, and be put into the family of an aunt or an uncle or a grandparent. Then the committee could send the money to the family member to help take care of the child.

Each day I helped translate about thirty applications into French. The way I did it was to look at the picture of the child. I did not read the application, I just took time to look at the picture of the child. Usually after only thirty or forty seconds, I became one with the child. I don't know how or why, but it's always like that. Then I could pick up the pen and translate the words from the application onto another sheet. Afterwards I realized that it was not me who had translated the application; it was the child and me, who had become one. Looking at his face or her face, I got motivated and I became him and he became me, and together we did the translation. It is very natural. You don't have to practice a lot of meditation to be able to do that. You just look, you allow yourself to be, and then you lose yourself in the child, and the child in you. This is one example which illustrates the way of perception recommended by the Buddha. In order to understand something, you have to be one with that something.

—*Thich Nhat Hanh, from* Being Peace

ONE HUNDRED ARMS OF COMPASSION

In Buddhism we have different images and symbols. One of my favorites is Kannon, the image of compassion. Kannon can be a male or a female. There are different physical images of Kannon, but one shows Kannon with many, many arms. Why does Kannon have so many arms? I believe it is because when Kannon took the vow to make peace among all sentient beings she was so overwhelmed by the enormity of what that meant that she burst apart into millions of pieces. But the energy of that same vow bought all those pieces back in the shape of a million arms. Each arm holds something different. One arm holds a watch, one holds glasses, one arm bears a pen, one a hoe, one arm a Christmas bag, one a condom. Each arm has something different for the proper occasion.

Each of us is an arm of Kannon, enabling Kannon to do her work. Like her, we're also overwhelmed, but when we realize that the millions of pieces are all operating as one, then there's no problem. The reason we get overwhelmed is that we're attached to a certain result or that we want to achieve a certain result or that we want to achieve a certain goal. If we weren't attached we wouldn't be overwhelmed. It's endless. And we just take one step after the next.

—*Bernard Glassman, from* Bearing Witness

GENEROSITY WITHOUT BOUNDS

Yeshe Tsogyal was the main disciple and consort of the great Tibetan master Padmasambhava, who is credited with bringing Buddhism to Tibet more than 1,200 years ago. Considered to be a reincarnation of the goddess Sarasvati, Yeshe Tsogyal was rumored to be so beautiful that by the time she was twelve years old, suitors from all the surrounding regions came to court her. After achieving great realization under the tutelage of Padmasambhava, who entrusted her with all the highest tantric teachings, she devoted her life to helping others, often undergoing incredible hardships to fulfill her vows. The following passage is taken from the biography of her life, compiled from an oral translation by Tarthang Tulku.

Tsogyal took upon herself the sufferings of others. . . . She gave her body to wild animals, clothing to those who were cold and food to the hungry. To the sick she gave medicine, to the poor riches. To the powerless, she gave protection, and to those with great desire, she gave her own body. She gave of her body and life in whatever manner would be of use to other beings. Without regard for herself, she even gave her own sense organs where they could be of use. . . .

Once. . . three men approached her carrying a cripple. She asked what had happened, and they explained: "We have come from 'On-phu in Tibet. The king ordered this man punished by having his kneecaps removed. A great and learned Tibetan told us that only the kneecaps of a woman could help him, otherwise there is no hope. Lady, it is said that you will give anything to those who have need. Thus, we have come to you. Could you possibly give us what we ask for?"

Looking at the cripple, Tsogyal saw the long, oblong scars on his legs and felt great compassion arise within her heart. "You may take from me whatever you need," she told them, "for I promised my teacher always to act for the benefit of beings by my body, speech, and mind."

So they took out a knife. "We need to make great incisions in your body. It will be very painful. . . . Can you stand it?"

"Whatever must happen, let it happen," she replied.

First, they cut across the top of the knee and then pulled out the knee caps with a loud popping noise. When they set the red objects down in front of Tsogyal for a moment she lost her breath. But she recovered and told the men to take them. They rejoiced and left. After a time, her knees healed.

LIBERATING BEINGS

Yuan Ch'i Beng of Hang Jou Province made a vow in his youth that he would always liberate the living. He was particularly fond of liberating mussels, clams, roe, and the like, for it didn't take much money to ransom these small sea creatures and so in one outing he could set free many lives. He also encouraged others to do likewise. In the year 1680, while at sea, the ship he was on ran into some reefs and capsized. Strangely enough, however, water did not seep into the vessel at all. Floating on its side, the ship finally reached safety, where it was discovered that several tens of thousands of little fishes, clams and mussels had congregated beneath the ship, keeping it afloat so that the water could not enter and sink it. Yuan understood that these must be the sea creatures that he had set free—that they had come to repay the debt of kindness and save his life in turn.

—*From* Cherishing Life, *edited by*
Bhikshuni Heng Ming and Upasika Kuo Tsai Round

CIRCLE OF LIFE

It is said in the Buddhist teachings that the practice of saving sentient beings from death creates enormous merit for this life and the next; it is still carried on today, particularly by Tibetan Buddhists. The Tibetan master Kusum Lingpa yearly releases brine shrimp into the ocean, most recently in Long Island Sound. The following story by an eyewitness records the buying and freeing of animals that marked the visit of the great Tibetan master Kyabje Trulshik Rinpoche to Brittany.

On the first of December 1999, at the urging of the Tibetan lama Pema Wangyal Rinpoche, all the crabs, spider crabs, lobsters, prawns, and cockles in the fish tanks of the supermarket in Penvenan, a small village in the north of Brittany, were bought so that they could blessed and put back in the sea. And as if that wasn't enough, to this already astonishing quantity were added many winkles, mussels, and scallops, and still more crabs, spider crabs, and lobsters from the wholesalers along the coast. About a dozen large crates were spread out in front of the house at Kerjoly, where Kyabje Trulshik Rinpoche had been invited to stay, and he and his monks were able to scrutinize a whole variety of marine life. Asking the names of each of the species, Rinpoche blessed each of the creatures individually. We then set off to a secluded and rocky part of the coast. When we arrived, the three Tibetan lamas and two monks organized a fishing party in reverse! With their pincers untied, the lobsters were put back in the sea, glad no doubt to be back in their watery element.

Watching, participating, we could only feel like the animals—fragile, liberated and protected—just like them.

—*Anonymous*

AUSPICIOUS ENCOUNTERS

It was my first day as a chaplain intern at a New York City hospital and I was terrified. My fellow students and I had received very little preparatory training and were basically told to sink or swim. Before meeting my first patient, I prayed deeply that I would be of benefit to someone, but I had doubts. Although I was an ordained interfaith minister, I had been brought up as a devout Reform Jew and my adult spiritual practice had been generally Buddhist. I wasn't sure how to pray with Christian patients and frankly, I wasn't even sure whether I could minister to Jewish patients, particularly the Orthodox ones who seemed to populate the hospital. Though I wasn't expecting to run into any Buddhists, at least my meditation practice had taught me that the most important thing I could do with a suffering person was to listen. Mostly, though, I wanted a sign that indeed my masters were guiding me.

After frittering away several hours reading patients' charts, I steeled myself to enter the first room. My first two patients were not very sick and were in fact eager to talk to a chaplain. But the third room! As I tentatively opened the door slowly I noticed a very handsome Latino face. And then my eyes moved down the sheets—a motorcycle accident had left him enclosed in full-body cast, neck to toes. I gulped, afraid to disturb him. After I introduced myself as an interfaith minister, I was surprised to see him looking deeply into my eyes. Then he said, "Well, then maybe *you* would know. What's that place between heaven and earth?"

I was shocked. There had been no preamble to this question. And being a novice chaplain, I had taken for granted he was Catholic. The only way I could answer this question was definitely not Catholic.

"Well, uh . . .," I stammered, "I do know about a place like that, but it's in the Tibetan Buddhist tradition. It's called the *bardo*—"

"Yes! That's it! The *barrrr*-do," he cried, excitedly, drawing out the r's with his Spanish accent.

"And who's that *rrr-rinpoche?*"

My mind stopped for a minute. There were hundreds of rinpoches, teachers in the Tibetan tradition.

You know," he said, getting adamant, "the one who wrote the *book!*"

My thoughts were spinning. There were hundreds of books.

But . . . wait . . . could he mean . . . Sogyal Rinpoche? One of *my* teachers? "You mean the one who wrote *The Tibetan Book of Living and Dying*?" I said.

"Yes, that's the one!" he said, enormously delighted.

I couldn't believe it. How was it that I was in a New York City hospital on my first day as a chaplain and I was talking about the bardo? Then, my few ministerial skills kicked in.

"I'm just wondering . . . why would you bring this up now?" I ventured. "I mean, what is your interest in the bardo?"

He held my gaze tightly, as if he had been waiting for just the right person to say this to.

"Because . . ." he said, drawing his words out slowly, "three days ago . . . I was . . . *there*."

What a strange thing to say. Generally, being in the bardo is an after-death experience. Now I caught him looking at me even more intently, and it was the first time I noticed just how shiny his eyes were—streaming light, in fact, as if he had been on a meditation retreat for a year. I had rarely seen those kind of eyes before, and usually only on the face of a great master.

Who *was* this man?

For a moment, we just looked at each other, perhaps in our own bardo, of not-here, not-there. There was so much I wanted to ask him, so much I wanted to know. Perhaps he had had an amazing near-death experience. I felt we could have gone on talking forever. But suddenly our connection was snapped. A beautiful young Indian woman, his wife, came in carrying his dinner. The conversation changed to social niceties. A technician came to take his blood. Soon it was my cue to leave. I promised to return as soon as I could.

All week I waited expectantly to return to my shift, but when I went to his room, I found his bed vacant. At first I had the sinking feeling he had died, but soon discovered that despite his massive injuries, he had been discharged a few days before. Somehow I felt cheated. When I returned to the chaplain's office, I discovered that he had been trying desperately to reach me all week, had even left several messages that had never gotten to me. Against all hospital rules, I hunted down his home address and wrote him a short note wishing him well and extended an invitation to contact me. But he never did.

Yet he had given me such a blessing. Though I felt I had done little to heal him, he had brought me immense healing—a young novice chaplain, afraid to talk to patients, fearful she would meet no one who spoke her "language." And then to have the most unexpected messenger, swathed in a body cast, invoking the name of my Tibetan teacher, reciting the title of his book, and embodying the power of the teaching of impermanence—well, it seemed only right that he would then disappear.

—*Pamela Bloom*

> All the buddhas, bodhisattvas, and enlightened beings are present at all moments to help us, and it is through the presence of the master that all of their blessings are focused directly at us.
>
> —*Sogyal Rinpoche*

NO GREATER LOVE

When I was three or four years old, Jamyang Khyentse Chökyi Lodrö, one of the great Tibetan masters of the past century, came to our village in Eastern Tibet on a pilgrimage because there were a lot of sacred caves in the area. When my family and I went to visit him, he bestowed upon me my present name and told my mother in private to take care of me because one day I might become of great benefit to others. As such, my family thought I should go to a monastery. I also had the feeling from a very young age that I wanted to be a monk. My mother used to tell me stories about how I would dress up in robes at the age of two and do lama dances [spontaneous sacred dancing done only by masters]. After we left Tibet and I was enrolled in the Darjeeling School in India, a very high lama came to my class one day and asked who wanted to be a monk. I ran right up to the front without any hesitation.

I began my Buddhist studies at around fifteen years of age. In the next two or three years I often heard the teaching that you should treat every sentient being as your parent, but to tell you the truth I didn't have any feeling for it. It was only a concept until one day when I heard the following story.

Before he became a master, Khenpo Shenga was a bandit who had spent his whole life, up to the time he was about thirty-five years old, robbing and killing people. One day he incurred the wrath of another group of bandits, who wanted his head and began to chase him. Running beside the horse he was escaping on was his beloved, beautiful mare, who also happened to have a baby growing in her stomach. Because she was pregnant she couldn't run fast, and although he loved the horse very much, his pride simply would not allow this beautiful specimen of a horse to fall into the hands of other bandits. So making a critical decision, he whipped out his sword and hit the mare on the backside, practically slicing her in two. She fell to the ground, stricken, and the baby horse came out. But even though the mare was practically in two pieces, still she was moving her head toward her prematurely born baby to see if it was all right. At that moment, Khenpo Shenga deeply grasped what it meant to be a parent, what it meant to be a mother, and his heart cracked open. On the spot he abandoned his wild ways and went off to look for a master. It is said that after this he then just skated through the practices and evolved quickly into a very great master who came to benefit many others.

When I heard this story it touched me deeply. It helped me understand what it means to recognize that all sentient beings have been your mother in some lifetime and how much gratitude one must feel for the love and affection they have given you. Like Khenpo Shenga, I saw that no matter how much suffering a mother goes through, still, the inclination to take care of one's baby is so deep, so ingrained into her being. Therefore it makes great sense to work for the benefit of all beings and treat them all as your parent. In its humble way this story completely changed my life and practice.

—*Khenpo Tsewang Gyatso*

> The more helpless beings are, the more it is your true nature to love them.
>
> —*His Holiness the Dalai Lama*

TRANSFORMATIVE FORGIVENESS

In the early 1990s, in Boston, Massachusetts, I met on occasion with a Vietnamese Buddhist sangha. Their temple was near a large, beige-brick housing development, and what had once been a basketball court for the neighboring housing development was their parking lot. One day their offices were broken into, a computer was stolen, and their temple was vandalized. A leader of the Vietnamese sangha was interviewed on television. As he gazed steadily into the camera he said simply, "I am trying to look more deeply, to understand why these people came and stole from us. Yes, I would like our computer back. But mostly, I wish to speak with the thieves, to see if there is something that we have done. Perhaps they want their basketball court back."

His compassionate attitude had an amazing ripple effect in the community. His looking deeply opened a way beyond crime and punishment, beyond violation and retribution. It was amazing to see him speaking like this on the evening news. The leader eventually did talk with the young men who broke into the Vietnamese temple, and the computer was returned. The community did not press criminal charges. Instead, they arranged for the young men to have access to their basketball court part of the time.

—*Kate O'Neill, from* Buddhist Women on the Edge

> Living a truly ethical life in which we look to putting the needs of others first, and providing for their happiness, has tremendous implications for our society. If we change internally—disarm ourselves by cutting to the root of our negative emotions—we can literally change the world.
>
> —*His Holiness the Dalai Lama*

LAMP IN THE DARK

Two years before he died when the plane he was piloting crashed in the Atlantic Ocean, John F. Kennedy, Jr. interviewed His Holiness the Dalai Lama. The interview appeared in the December 1997 issue of *George,* the magazine

Kennedy founded. In the "Editor's Letter" of that issue, he described his visit to Dharamsala, the home of the Tibetan government in exile.

At precisely 8 A.M. on the morning of the anniversary of Mahatma Gandhi's 128th birthday, the Dalai Lama burst into a large receiving room filled with golden Buddhist statues and tangkas. Beneath his maroon-colored robes he wore a pair of brown oxfords, the kind that English schoolboys wear, and olive-colored socks. Though his English is halting, his eyes, which peer over wire-rimmed glasses, are astonishingly mirthful and expressive. As he greeted me, he took my bandaged hand and, instead of recoiling—as many did for fear of hurting me—held it in both of his hands, rubbing and patting it vigorously. It didn't hurt. . . .

A combination of joy and thoughtfulness is the source of the Dalai Lama's considerable personal charisma. Though he has shared in the deprivation and humiliation of the larger community he rules, his presence is not at all grave. As someone once described the Dalai Lama, "You are not overwhelmed by him when he's seated in front of you, but when you look away his presence fills up the whole room."

As a foreigner and a democrat (small d), I have a natural inclination toward skepticism and wanted to find the point where the image of infallibility ends and the human being begins. But it's not easy to do. The Dalai Lama has spent a lifetime and (if you subscribe to the Buddhist beliefs, countless lifetimes), learning to accept himself and his circumstances. It shows. The experience of meeting and talking with him is not like interviewing an American politician: There's no voting record to challenge, no brewing scandal, no gaffe from the past. How do you maintain your skepticism in the face of a man who says that what he'd most like to do if he had time off is spend those years solely alone, in solitary contemplation?

At the precise moment that our allotted time was up we said our goodbyes and he bustled out of the door and ducked under an umbrella to escape the late-monsoon rain that had just begun. I watched until the small entourage disappeared down the hill and I smiled at the few aides who remained in the room. We were content but oddly deflated. It was as if we were all in a dark room and the fellow with the lantern had just left.

—John F. Kennedy, Jr.

LIVING BEAUTY

When I began to study a spiritual form of Japanese flower-arranging called Ikebana-Sangetsu, I discovered I was slowly developing a deeper understanding of the connection between all life. In our first class, my teacher said that flowers can actually talk, that they each have their own way of being beautiful. They have *prana,* life force, so you have to pay full attention to them, rather than imposing your own ideas of beauty on them. So I began to ask the flowers how *they* wanted to be arranged, what positioning would make them feel most beautiful, and I waited and listened. Even after they had been set in the vase, I would discover sometimes that in the morning they had rearranged themselves during the night. Even though they were secured in the vase, they always seemed to be minutely straining to find their right place. At the same time, they were not fully independent; they needed loving care. They were dependent on me, or whomever their caretaker was for the day, to water them, to keep them moist. Sometimes I would watch other people spraying water on the arrangements and I would feel so moved. The droplets left on the green petals and flower buds seemed to be dewdrops of compassion, so delicately poised, touching the source of life, nourishing the heart of beauty. This experience made me feel how simple it could be, if our minds and hearts are set in the right way, to water not only plants, but human beings—to treat all living creatures in a way that allows them their right to be beautiful, in their own space and time.

What we came to notice in our class was that flowers could also listen. Our teacher urged us to always remind the flowers when we passed how beautiful they were and to thank them for sharing that beauty with us. When we did this, when we made our arrangements with this kind of love and devotion, we always found that the flowers remained beautiful and fresh for many more days than expected.

—*Pamela Bloom*

CANINE COMPASSION

He came to me in the dead of winter, Christmas Day. Someone tied him up with a thin rope to a pole in front of Dudley's Paw, a local pet food store. It was snowing and he sat there calmly, patiently waiting in the cold. Since it was Christmas Day and no stores were open, I couldn't imagine someone had tied him up while they went shopping. Nevertheless, I left a note "If you left your dog here, please call. . ." with my phone number. No one called.

Not new to encounters with abandoned dogs, I approached carefully and spoke gently in an attempt to assure him no harm was meant. Then I untied him and brought him home. Ginger, a retriever/border collie and Fonzie, a husky, my two resident companion animals, protested as I brought the intruder into the house. I felt it was safer to put him in the bedroom so he could warm up and be safe from the howling and barking of two jealous dogs.

I soon learned from his behavior that Barney had been a trained attack dog, mistrustful of most people but particularly of men. He had scars on his face and was in dreadful condition.

My life soon changed in every aspect. I couldn't have friends visit because to him they were strangers and posed a threat. Barney caught me unaware a few times while I was walking him and he bit a few unsuspecting people. His worst bite was the veterinary doctor who first examined him the day after his rescue. The doctor wanted to decapitate him to determine if he was rabid since there are no medical tests to determine this condition. The fight to save his life began with my calling the entire animal rescue community. After much begging and talking, the vet agreed to release Barney to the Center for Animal Care and Control for ten days of observation for rabid behavior, a New York City law for all dogs who have bitten and do not have proof of rabies inoculation.

After ten days the C.A.C.C. released Barney back to me with a clean bill of health as far as rabies was concerned, but his emotional and physical condition had worsened.

I had to build a steel grid separation to keep Barney and Fonzie from killing each other. The two males fought bitterly for a year and a half, running up and down the grid and biting fiercely at the steel squares. When they weren't madly barking, growling, biting, and baring teeth, they were watching every movement, every nuance of the other.

As I watched Barney and Fonzie spending hours watching each other, I felt that in time they would understand and through this understanding be able to live together without a steel grid between them. I knew this way of life—forced separation, constant fighting—couldn't be good for anyone.

Even though I'd been rescuing dogs for many years, I was at a loss as to how to approach socializing these two macho male dogs, so I invited trainers to give me some assistance. Every trainer assured me what I was attempting was a lost cause and suggested I get Barney another home, as if homes for difficult dogs were so plentiful! I simply would not accept this.

There is a Tibetan Buddhist verse called "The Song of the Profound View" by Geshe Robten that goes like this: "When I examined this old monk who previously seemed so existent, he turned out to be just like tracks of a bird in the sky. The appearance of a bird just turns through the mind, but if one looks for her tracks, they are inexpressible: emptiness is all there is."

So if this were true, then Barney or Fonzie could not be characterized by their actions. I was sure that with training and generation of compassion, the goal of mutual respect could be achieved. But how to go about it?

Meditation.

Each day I'd go into Barney's fourteen-by-six-foot enclosure and spend time reading and talking to him. I also rubbed his chest, an established way to soothe a male dog. Then I'd go into Fonzie's "territory" and do the same with Ginger and Fonzie. I would also meditate and do yoga in what I felt was neutral space where Barney, Fonzie, and Ginger could watch.

On walks I worked with Barney, teaching him "sit" and "down" commands, which gave him some direction and created a sense of safety.

All this time, I had to walk Barney separately, which involved setting up gates so that I could get him out of his enclosure without any bloody encounters between Fonzie and Barney. Once or twice I had been too hasty in closing the gate and they did "lock horns." Another time Fonzie was badly bitten by Barney above his eye. So to save him from further damage, the next time they got close to one another, I put my body in between, receiving a hefty bite on my left thigh from Fonzie, who had lived with me for fifteen years! But in the wild state of madness, fear, and aggression, he didn't recognize me so I could not fault him. Barney, however, was very aware of me and at my "Sit!" command, he backed off.

After a year and a half of separate walks, separate living spaces, and much anxiety, one day something within my heart said that this was the day to attempt a walk with all three dogs. Heart pounding, I leashed up Fonzie and Ginger, then opened the door to Barney's enclosure. I watched every hair on both male dogs for any sign of sudden explosion. Nothing.

We carefully walked out together, as I spoke reassuringly all the while, "Good Fonzie, good Barney." From then on, though the two never really played together, their mutual tolerance was something I could depend upon. Ultimately I was able to go to work and leave all three dogs free to roam the apartment to their heart's content.

Watching Barney unfold like a lotus flower from being fearful, aggressive, angry, and mistrustful to wide-eyed, trusting, patient, obedient, and calm was a miraculous transformation.

—*Sharon Azar-Hahn*

If we are peaceful, if we are happy, we can blossom like a flower, and everyone in our family, our entire society, will benefit from our peace.

— *Thich Nhat Hanh*

SHARING PLEASURE

One day on retreat in the south of France, Sogyal Rinpoche suddenly had to leave to go to an emergency meeting in Paris. It was an abrupt departure, and we did not see him for several days. The retreat continued on without him, but many of us were severely disappointed. Some of us had come such a long way, and every moment in the teacher's presence seemed so precious. Finally he returned and he shared with us scenes from his trip, vividly painting a picture of the glowing fields and quaint country homes of the region between Montpelier in the south and Paris in the north. With his laughter and enthusiasm, Rinpoche had a way of speaking in such detail that it was not difficult to feel you were in the car with him.

And then he said quite humbly, "As I was driving through this region, staring out the window, there was a moment . . . a moment . . . I was so moved by the beauty and spaciousness of the landscape, that I found myself saying, 'May all beings enjoy such beauty. May all beings have the opportunity to enjoy such views in their lives.'"

By simply giving us a glimpse of his heart, Sogyal was trying to teach us that boundless generosity in which no experience, even the greatest bliss of enlightenment, is held for oneself. In that moment it was easy to see how genuine the feeling was for him, how natural such a human response could be, if we allowed it. In a way that I only see now, it was not too different from how my own mother is, always wanting to share whatever good bit of food or trinket or gift she has with me. From that moment on, I've tried to remember to share with others whatever experiences of beauty and pleasure I had—even if only through silent aspiration. But it hasn't always been easy. How many times do we become so involved in eating an ice cream cone, laughing at a great joke, hearing beautiful music that we wipe out the awareness that there is anything else in the world but our own personal pleasure. But slowly, as I tried to train myself to remember and "share," I noticed something in me start to open and soften, to expand. Slowly the exercise began to take on a life of its own and became joy. And it certainly made any experience of happiness that much more profound by wishing it for all.

—*Pamela Bloom*

THE BULLET THAT STOPS ALL WARS

Chân Không is a Buddhist nun who was one of the first four clergy ordained by Vietnamese master Thich Nhat Hanh. During the Vietnam War she was a forerunner in social welfare programs before becoming an international advocate of peace. Her memoir of her early days in Vietnam during the sixties and seventies, from which this story is taken, is one of the most searing records of physical and spiritual warriorship ever written.

One night, we stopped in Son Khuong, a remote village where the fighting was especially fierce. As we were about to go to sleep in our boat, we suddenly heard shooting, then screaming, then shooting again. The young people in our group were seized with panic, and a few young men jumped into the river to avoid the bullets. I sat quietly in the boat with two nuns and breathed consciously to calm myself. Seeing us so calm, everyone stopped panicking, and we quietly chanted *The Heart Sutra,* concentrating deeply on this powerful chant. For a while, we didn't hear any bullets. I don't know if they actually stopped or not. The day after, I shared my strong belief with my co-workers. "When we work to help people, the bullets have to avoid us, because we can never avoid the bullets. When we have good will and great love, when our only aim is to help those in distress, I believe there is a kind of magnetism, the energy of goodness, that protects us from being hit by the bullets. We only need to be serene. Then, even if a bullet hits us, we can accept it calmly, knowing that everyone has to die one day. If we die in service, we can die with a smile, without fear."

—*Ven. Chân Không, from* Learning True Love

TRANSFORMING EVIL

Palden Gyatso is a Tibetan monk who has spent more than thirty years in Chinese prisons, longer than any other Tibetan political prisoner. The tortures that he underwent have been shared by many of his fellow compatriots. He was assigned to till the prison fields yoked to a plow like an ox. On days when he was too exhausted to pull the plow, he was kicked and beaten for insubordination. In summer he and fellow prisoners were chained to the ceiling, a fire built beneath them, while in winter they were doused with freezing water. Through it all, it was only his meditation practice that gave him strength.

I am not a learned Buddhist scholar and during my years in prison I was not allowed to engage in formal practice. But I had the background knowledge and I practiced within. [When I was in jail] I had boiling water poured on me by a guard because he didn't like my attitude, and no medical treatment was given to me afterward. Another guard jabbed me all over, including in my mouth, with an electric cattle prod. When I regained consciousness, most of my teeth were gone. . . . I would meditate on Tonglen when they gave me electric shocks. Normally the body is gripped by convulsions, but I often felt the electricity as just something cold. This is how I survived—

by putting more energy into my interior practice and transforming negativity into benefit.

—*Palden Gyatso, from the* Snow Lion *newsletter*

FERRY OF COMPASSION

I needed some part-time work to do while I was painting, something that wouldn't interfere with it and at the same time would contain the energy of the sacred art I was doing. I looked in the paper and saw that schoolbus drivers were needed. It was in the summer and a month before school was to start, so it seemed like a good idea. When I arrived for the interview, Chester, the man who would become my supervisor, said, "Well, let's see first how you do in a van," and took me right out on the road. We were driving around the reservoir of our county, which is a very beautiful and special place, and he started talking about what it means to be a bus driver. I remember him saying, "We don't get much respect because we don't make a lot of money. But except for maybe the parents, there is nobody who cares more about the kids than we do—about their safety, how they *are.*"

It really moved me to hear this. Imagine—this was a very humble man, with dirt on his hands, wearing that old mechanic's uniform, a middle-aged man for whom the sun rose and set on his family. As I worked for him over many months I came to realize that his gentleness and love for all of us, from the bus drivers to the kids, set the tone for the whole business. Sometimes he would even apologize that he couldn't pay us more. And whenever there was a hassle with the school system, he was always behind us. One time when I had stood up for the wrong person out of ignorance and had been betrayed, Chester and I had a big talk in his office about credibility. "How can we do any work in the world without credibility?" he said. "You can't work with people unless they believe in you. And when people complain about 'society,' don't they get it? We *are* the society. If we don't stand up for the kids, who will?" It was something in the way he said it that always stuck with me. For him being a bus driver *was* his spiritual practice.

This became true for me as well. I remember one little girl who had a lot of behavioral problems. She hadn't been allowed on another bus because she had bitten the driver and had hit the other children. She had even acted out at school and was becoming a danger to others. When she first came on the bus I had the monitor take care of her, but somehow she just got wedged in, blocked off from the other children. Watching her staring out the window, all alone, I felt she needed to integrate herself on the bus. By this time I knew the kids on my bus—we had really nice ones—and part of the ride is to get along with each other, to join the party because the kids do things together—they have raffles, they draw. It's like a little happening.

Melody was always the last one I picked up, so I spoke to the other kids first as they got on. I explained how Melody ought to be sitting with someone because she's really shy, and to my surprise, they all volunteered. One day, when the monitor wasn't available, one little girl in particular, a second-grader, just started entertaining her. She had a paper Santa Claus and was doing a very funny ventriloquism act with it and had everybody, including Melody, laughing. She'd say in Santa's voice, "Oh, mind if I sit here? Ho ho ho, I got a list and I'm checking it twice. Oh, you're a good little girl—too good to be true. You're as good as gold." After that, she'd ask, "Can I sit with Melody today? Is today the day?" And what happened is that this little troubled girl became ecstatic. She said to me, "My mother will be so proud of me, I have a new friend on the bus now and all the other kids want to sit with me." I didn't feel I did anything myself, I only set the stage, but it took only a week for this troubled child to become a totally different kid.

—*Julia Russell*

> Education is much more than a matter of imparting the knowledge and skills by which narrow goals are achieved. It is also about opening the child's eyes to the needs and rights of others.
>
> — *His Holiness the Dalai Lama*

PACIFYING AGGRESSION

Dilgo Khyentse Rinpoche was one of the greatest Tibetan masters of the twentieth century, a luminescent mountain of a man who physically towered over Tibetans and Westerners alike, yet deeply imbued each one he met with the poetic eloquence of his scholarship, the spaciousness of his mind, and the warmth of his near-saintly compassion. As Thondup Tulku relates in his book *Masters of Meditation and Miracles,* Khyentse Rinpoche eschewed flying on his last trip right before his death, just to make the journey between Bhutan and Kalimpong, India, by car so that he might visit with an old disciple, despite the toll the arduous travel would make on his health. In a life that lasted eighty years, he spent over twenty of them in retreat, and though he would never admit to it, his spiritual powers were vast; even his wife claimed to often see strange lights emanating from his meditation hut. Below is a description of yet another example of the power of his blessing.

One of Dilgo Khyentse Rinpoche's nephews often went hunting, and he owned a celebrated gun. When it happened that Khyentse Rinpoche visited their house one day, his sister and nephew's mother told him, "This gun has killed so many animals, please bless it." Khyentse Rinpoche put the gun to his mouth and blew into it. It never fired again. After that, whenever Khyentse Rinpoche visited they all hid their guns. At the same house, there was a huge dog, which had killed many goats, and the family asked him to bless the dog. Khyentse Rinpoche took the ball of tsampa he was eating at the time, blew on it and then gave it to the dog. The dog ate it, and never went out of the house again.

—*Orgyen Tobgyal Rinpoche*

CURING OFFICE RAGE

I work as an Internet producer and have a superior in my company who simply despises me. In fact, I was thinking about quitting my job because he is so rough on me. My husband, who is a very strong meditator, told me I should consider this guy my teacher since he was giving me a great opportunity to develop patience and compassion. So I decided to bite the bullet and stay.

Recently the two of us had a showdown that turned into an interdepartmental war. Before I began Buddhist practice I would have tried to outwit him, beat him at his game somehow. But since becoming involved in Buddhism, I tried to see if I could calm my own emotions by practicing Tonglen, the meditation practice in which one breathes in the suffering of the environment and breathes out compassion. Because it is such a subtle practice, nobody knew I was even doing it. After a lot of angry words had been tossed about, somebody finally suggested, "Why don't we go around the table and say what it would take for all of us to get along?" For some reason I had to talk first and I didn't have a clue what to say, but suddenly this came out of me: "You know, it's not about writing a memo, it's not about a meeting, it's something much more intangible, like coming into each other's office and leaving the work stuff on the side and just talking on a human level because we all essentially want the same thing. We want the project to be successful, we want a happy environment, we just need to drop our animosity toward each other." Suddenly to everybody's surprise this officer who despised me started talking about his *mother*—how they hadn't spoken in ten years and how they were now in relationship therapy together. We were all quite shocked, but I just kept looking at him and practiced compassion. It's clear to me now that the atmosphere changed in the room simply because I wasn't reverting to my normal hostile reaction.

It also helped for me to think of the situation as impermanent. I remember telling myself, he is not forever, I am not forever, nothing here is forever. Instead, here's an opportunity to make this moment mean something for myself and for my colleagues, rather than hanging onto a position of combat. At the end of the meeting, one of the accountants started teasing everybody saying, "Oh, I love you guys," as if to make fun of the situation, but it really did describe the place we had all gotten to. What's amazing is that these are not people who are into emotions at all; they are into demographics.

—*Anonymous*

Loving-kindness for oneself is the golden key to appreciating other people, even the ones that you drive you crazy.

— *Pema Chödrön*

SIMPLE CARE

I was in a bad car accident in the late seventies. I arrived at Insight Meditation Society on crutches to teach a long retreat and I was having difficulty getting around. That was the year His Holiness the Dalai Lama came to visit. The preparations for his visit were intensive because we had to arrange a great deal of security for this man who is considered a head of state. Our peaceful, rural retreat center became a stronghold. Pleasant Street was barricaded off, and state policemen patrolled the roof with guns. There were video cameras and a lot of excited activity. I was feeling dismal on crutches, especially when I ended up in the back of the huge crowd waiting to greet the Dalai Lama when he arrived. The car with His Holiness in it pulled up at last and was greeted by the cameras, the people and the armed policemen. The Dalai Lama got out, looked around and saw me standing way in the back of the room, leaning on the crutches.

He cut straight through the crowd and came up to me, as though he were homing in on the deepest suffering in the situation. He took my hand, looked me in the eye and asked, "What happened?"

It was a beautiful moment. I had been feeling so left out. Now I suddenly felt cared for. The Dalai Lama did not have to make the pain go away; in fact he could not. But his simple acknowledgment, his openness, helped me feel included. Every act can be expressive of our deepest values.

—*Sharon Salzberg, from* Lovingkindness

> If you were to ask me 'What is the essence of Buddhism?' I would answer that it's to awaken. And the function of that awakening is learning how to serve.
>
> —*Bernard Glassman*

LOVE WITHOUT BIAS

Ten or fifteen years ago, I was living in a very small space in Paris, and every night I walked my dog outside for about an hour. Many times we'd go to a little garden near the Champs

Élysées and I would meditate there, at the same time watching and playing with my dog. The garden was about one hundred feet from the Champs Élysées, and even though there were a lot of people walking past, they didn't see me, so I felt I could be alone. I remember thinking about my teachers. They used to say how important it is to feel compassion for everybody without judgment or favoritism, so one evening I decided to try. The people walking by were close enough to see, but too far away for me to have any thought about them. So I began to pray completely freely for these people without judgment. Everybody was a stranger, but at the same time I felt very close to them because I could really give all my love very freely, without thinking about receiving anything in return. Suddenly I was completely surrounded by bliss. I was giving love, but in return I was feeling ten times more. I was really receiving the blessing and compassion of my masters.

Often I would do the same thing in the car. Sometimes we'd get stuck in the car in traffic or be waiting for a light, and my eyes would meet someone for maybe a fraction of a second in the street. In that moment, very often I would just try looking at the person, smiling and sending my love, feeling in my heart, I love you, for example. Looking at the person and smiling at him or her without thinking was very easy because it was just a momentary glance as the person is passing by. So my love was much more like equanimity—all-inclusive, without bias. Sometimes I could really see that the person would be completely transformed by this kind of shock—that somebody was smiling at him or her for no reason.

—*Michel Rousseau*

When you begin to touch your heart or let your heart be touched, you begin to discover that it's bottomless, that it doesn't have any resolution, that this heart is huge, vast, and limitless. You begin to discover how much warmth and gentleness is there, as well as how much space.

—*Pema Chödrön*

TRANSFORMING ANGER

More than twenty-five years ago, Pema Chödrön was ordained as a Buddhist nun in the Kagyu lineage of Tibetan Buddhism. Today as Abbess of Gampo Abbey in Nova Scotia, she is known for the mixture of brutal self-honesty and kitchen-sink compassion that she brings to her teaching.

I recently received a letter from a friend in which she dumped all over me and told me off. My first reaction was to be hurt and my second reaction was to get mad, and then I began to compose this letter in my mind, this very dharmic letter that I was going to write back to her using all the teachings . . . to tell her off. Because of the style of our relationship, she would have been intimidated by a dharmic letter, but it wouldn't have helped anything. It would have further forced us into these roles of being two separate people, each of us believing in our roles more and more seriously, that I was the one who knew it all and she was the poor student. But on that day when I had spent so much energy composing this letter, just by a turn of circumstance, something happened to me that caused me to feel tremendous loneliness. I felt sad and vulnerable. In that state of mind, I suddenly knew where my friend's letter had come from—loneliness and feeling left out. It was her attempt to communicate.

Sometimes when you're feeling miserable, you challenge people to see if they will still like you when you show them how ugly you can get. Because of how I myself was feeling I knew that what she needed was not for somebody to dump back on her. So I wrote a very different letter from what I had planned, an extremely honest one that said, "You know, you can dump on me all you like and put all of your stuff out there, but I'm not going to give up on you." It wasn't a wishy-washy letter that avoided the issue that there had been a confrontation and that I had been hurt by it. On the other hand, it wasn't a letter in which I went to the other extreme and lashed out. For the first time, I felt I had experienced what it meant to exchange oneself for other. When you've been there you know what it feels like, and therefore you can give something that you know will open up the space and cause things to keep flowing. You can give something that will help someone else connect with their own insight and courage and gentleness, rather than further polarize the situation.

—*Pema Chödrön, from* Start Where You Are

Relative bodhichitta comes from the simple and basic experience of realizing that you could have a tender heart in any situation.

—*Chögyam Trungpa Rinpoche*

SILENT BLESSINGS

About eighteen years ago, I was staying at La Sonnerie in Dordogne, France, which was the French residence of His Holiness Dilgo Khyentse Rinpoche. People would come from all over the world to hear his teachings. He lived there for one or two months at a time. Often Khyentse Rinpoche would just start teaching or giving a transmission and anyone who was there had to come within minutes if they wanted to hear it. It didn't matter whether there were three or thirty people—if the teachings were flowing he would just teach. The primary purpose was to give transmissions to the young tulkus and the students entering the three-year retreat, but of course the teaching was open to the others as well.

At the same time, Nyoshul Khenpo Rinpoche was also living there; he was teaching the students in three-year retreat. Back then, most people didn't know who he really was, a secret master, completely anonymous. He later became the teacher of Sogyal Rinpoche and others.

One day I was very sad because of difficulty with a relationship and I was sitting on the grass crying. Nyoshul Khenpo Rinpoche saw me and came over and sat down beside me on the grass. Khenpo Rinpoche could only speak by whispering—and he couldn't speak French or English at all. Even so, he talked to me through hand signs, whispering, and mimicking. I remember he was waving his arms around and blowing with his lips to indicate how big and spacious the sky was, and he pointed to his smile to indicate I should cheer up. He was so simple and it was all very clear, even though he was only using signs and facial expressions. He just sat down on the grass and opened my mind.

A few years later, I often drove him in my car to visit some students in retreat. My dog was often in the car and unfortunately had chewed up the seats, so the car was a real mess. But Khenpo Rinpoche just got in the car with the dog and was perfectly happy. It never mattered what the situation was. Once, on the way back he asked me to wait. We parked near a bluff that had a beautiful view, and we just sat there, looking at the sky and not talking. He was so simple, with absolutely no protocol. In fact, he was teaching me how to meditate. It was wonderful to have a master like that.

Sometimes when Nyoshul Khenpo Rinpoche was in Paris, he liked to be in the Métro, or in the street, because there he could see people in their ordinary lives. It would always amaze me that he could just go up to somebody and touch the material of their clothes very lightly, and it would never bother people because he was so natural, happy, and smiling. He was just spontaneously curious, a little bit like a child, about anything new and interesting, such as a new fabric. In fact, I think it was also his way to connect with people, and I'm sure they were receiving a blessing without even knowing it! He just had the ability to be everywhere and anywhere, with a look in his eyes always so full of compassion and kindness.

—*Michel Rousseau*

THE SUPREME EMOTION

On a trip to Europe, I took the opportunity to visit the site of the Nazi death camp at Auschwitz. Even though I had heard and read a great deal about the place, I found myself completely unprepared for the experience. My initial reaction to the sight of the ovens in which hundreds of thousands of human beings were burned was one of total revulsion. I was dumbfounded at the sheer calculation and detachment from feeling to which they bore horrifying testimony. Then, in the museum which forms part of the visitor centre, I saw a collection of shoes. A lot of them were patched or small, having obviously belonged to children and poor people. This saddened me particularly. What could *they* have possibly done, what harm? I stopped and prayed—moved profoundly both for the victims and for the perpetrators of this calamity—that such a thing would never happen again. And, in the knowledge that, just as we all have the capacity to act selflessly out of concern for others' well-being, so do we all have the potential to be murderers and torturers, I vowed to do all I could to ensure that nothing like this happened again.

—*His Holiness the Dalai Lama,*
from Ethics for the New Millennium

DYING INTO LOVE

When my mother became terminally ill, I went out to Las Vegas, where she was living, to take care of her. My mother was a very devout Catholic and raised us as devout Catholics. As I grew older, however, I became increasingly disaffected by certain perspectives of the Catholic Church but retained many positive values from my Christian experience as I explored other spiritual traditions, ultimately finding a home in Tibetan Buddhism. My mother, understandably, did not share my enthusiasm, and her disapproval was the source of some pain.

My mother loved people and loved to give service, but there was also a dark side to her. She was very complicated emotionally, and she acted out a lot of the trauma she had experienced as a child on my father, my sister, and myself. By the time she became ill, I was fortunate to have worked out most of my feelings toward her but still did not see a connection between her personal interactions and her attendance at daily Mass and the rosaries she said all the time. She had a very special connection with the Blessed Mother; in fact, she had Blessed Mothers all over the house, in the garage, in the garden, guarding her hat collection in the carport. I could never figure out, however, how could she be saying the rosary every day and be so awful at times.

My sister and I both had had hospice training, so by the time my mother was moving into active dying, we weren't afraid to be involved in the process. Inspired by Sogyal Rinpoche's teachings on death and dying in his book *The Tibetan Book of Living and Dying,* I wanted to help my mother have as good a death as possible. Every day I found myself dropping more and more of my judgmental mind and becoming more interested in supporting her to have confidence in her own object of devotion. Even when she could no longer talk, I wouldn't leave the room without reminding her of the Blessed Virgin's presence nearby. And then I would go into my room and pour over Rinpoche's book for guidance. One day, when it seemed to me my mother was especially suffering in her semicomatose state, I was inspired to read to her the chapter about what happens to the body when it dies and how to meditate at the time of death. To my surprise, I found myself naturally translating the Buddhist terms so my mother could understand their essence as Christian. But I was still of two minds: I'd meditate in my room with my mala [Buddhist prayer beads] and then go into my mother's room and say the rosary for her. Since I was staying alone in the house with her, I would check on her a couple of times a night, and at some point, I saw myself trying to manage the situation like some spiritual cowboy, with my mala in one hand and a rosary in the other, trying to meet both my spiritual needs and hers. In that moment when I was fervently saying "my" prayers and "her" prayers and "our" prayers, everything exploded, and any conceptual distinction between Buddhist and Catholic, between my mother and me, just dissolved. My mala became my rosary became my mala—in one seamless loving regard.

Prior to this, I thought I had reached a deep place of forgiveness for my mother, but in that moment, I realized something deeper—I did not want her to suffer at all anymore, no matter how much harm she had caused me or how much that harm might affect me in the future. And that became the dominant focus for me being with her until she died. Even my sister picked up on this energy and began behaving in the same way. Although my mother couldn't speak, we kept gently encouraging her to let go of anything she might be holding against us as we had already done for her. We continued to encourage her to focus on the Virgin Mary above her head, ready to receive and comfort her. We just wanted her to leave this life having complete faith in her own daily Christian practice.

In the moment she breathed her last breath on Mother's Day, she died very easily. We continued talking quietly to her, telling her she had now entered this odd but very natural process called death and encouraged her to keep connecting to the Blessed Mother. And we had total confidence this was helpful to her. In fact, it was so total and complete for us that to this day we are convinced that our mother had a blessed transition and that her death purified much of which she needed to address in this lifetime.

—*Michael Damian*

> Believe as you sit by the dying person that you are sitting by someone who has the potential to be a buddha. Imagine their buddha nature as a shining and stainless mirror, and all their pain and anxiety a thin, gray mist on it that can quickly clear. This will help you to see them as lovable and forgivable, and draw out of you your unconditional love; you will find this attitude will allow the dying person to open remarkably to you. . . . [But] remember, you can do nothing to inspire the person in front of you if you do not inspire yourself first.
>
> —*Sogyal Rinpoche*

PASSING ON THE LIGHT

I spent my late teens and half of my twenties as a gay man indulging in my newfound independence, searching in all the wrong places for what I know now to be philosophical truth, and hell-bent in the pursuit of parties and sexual gratification. Having grown up in a small American village, I had not known any other gay men as a child and so had no role models. Alcohol seemed to help me accept my sexuality and to give me courage and wild times. It also isolated me from my family and friends, ruined my self-esteem, and wreaked havoc with my job security. Luckily, I found a twelve-step program in my mid-twenties and sobered up.

Soon I started a serious relationship, came out to my family, got a job managing a restaurant, and returned to college to finish my degree. I even started running competitively. I was still young and life looked promising. What more could I ask for?

Then, in the late eighties and early nineties, AIDS started to rock our world. It was everywhere I turned. First, a few acquaintances, then a few friends, then many friends, then my significant other was diagnosed. Although AIDS was dominant in my life, I seemed able to contend with its ugly presence. That was until my own HIV diagnosis brought me to my knees.

Walking into the doctor's office, I thought I was prepared for anything. I had three years of sobriety and twelve-step programming under my belt. I couldn't have been more wrong. When I was told that I was positive, I stared at the wall in disbelief, tears streaming down my face. All I could think was, "I'M GOING TO DIE, I'M GOING TO DIE." When my friend Barbara hugged me, I sobbed deep inaudible cries and my body heaved in her arms. I had no idea where to turn or how to tell my family. For several days my mind was paralyzed, trying to sort and prioritize a meaningless life.

After living in a state of numbness for two months, I was fortunate to discover a wonderful support organization that existed at the time for people with life-challenging illness. It was called the Manhattan Center for Living and was founded by Marianne Williamson. I registered as a client and was struck by the fact that many of the clients were also volunteer staff members. After only two months, I was so inspired by helping others that I made a conscious decision to devote my life to doing service. In less than three months, I was asked to join the small paid staff. This gave me a tremendous opportunity to do everything from client counseling to managing the crisis center on weekends.

Watching people persevere against seemingly insurmountable odds with such positive and courageous attitudes provided me with a powerful example for my own life. But death still surrounded us. The first few struck me deeply to the core; to watch such beautiful lights dimmed in such an awful manner ripped my very being apart. Not knowing if I would literally see someone again, I began to treat everyone differently, more kindly and lovingly. I started to feel my heart open more and more.

Yet, as the death toll constantly increased, continuing to remain open and vulnerable became more and more difficult. After months and months of tragedies, deaths of friends no longer felt like a personal issue; grieving had been reduced to moving their file from the active file cabinet to the deceased file cabinet and posting a notice of their passing on the community bulletin board. During my last two months at the center, I lost one of my best friends and, unbelievably, about twenty other friends. I was completely paralyzed emotionally and didn't know what I was experiencing.

Emotionally burned out, I left the center and happened upon an ad for an HIV retreat at a Zen monastery. I realized I needed to spend time on my own healing. I joined the retreat and eventually decided to remain there in residence, first as a lay student, then as an ordained monk.

Over the next several years I found myself shedding many tears, especially in meditation. One day I was asked to organize the very same retreat for people with HIV and AIDS that had drawn me there in the first place. Strengthened now by my meditation practice, I found myself joyously hosting the weekend, gathering many different bodyworkers and healers, and cooking nourishing vegetarian food for the retreatants. It was a demanding schedule that afforded only four hours of sleep each night, but it was one that I completely gave myself to.

Recently an old friend found his way to the retreat as a bodyworker. Over the years since I had known him as a client at the Manhattan Center for Living, he had been developing his own healing skills and was just now beginning to give back to the AIDS community. When I asked him what his motivation had been, I was stunned. He told me that for many years he had watched me helping others and had been moved so much by my ceaseless giving that he had decided to devote his life in the same way with generosity, enthusiasm, and commitment. He even wanted to help me coordinate the next year's retreat. I was speechless, tears in my eyes, a lump in my throat.

To my mind, I had done nothing out of the ordinary; all those years I had only followed my aching heart. I myself had been inspired by others, but I never imagined that my conscious devotion to service would ever inspire another person so deeply as to give himself so totally in the same way. I was, and am, forever grateful.

—*Seppo Ed Farrey*

ALL-PERVADING KINDNESS

The Dalai Lama mentioned in a lecture in India in 1972 that all beings are always kind. Shortly after hearing this teaching, I visited the elder of the Dalai Lama's two tutors, a man who seemed to me the very incarnation of love. I asked him how it could be said that sentient beings are always only kind. He answered that all beings are kind because they are our field of merit—those in relation to whom we can practice helpful attitudes that empower our minds.

To my sight, he was a person who truly viewed beings this way. My impression that he possessed profound recognition of all sentient beings as extraordinarily valuable was so strong that it was almost painful to be in his presence. His magnanimity offended the part of my mind that wanted him to value me specially. I wanted him to think, "This is an intelligent person," or, "It is so nice to see this person." He did in fact appear to take great pleasure in seeing me; his attitude was neither neutral nor passive. Yet, I knew from his presence that his sense of joy would be equally great on seeing any other sentient being. He would recognize any particular positive or negative qualities, but he would not value people differently because of them. His valuation was based on something deeper than those qualities, and it was a marvelous teaching just to enter his presence because it required me to forsake a few baser qualities while I was there.

—*Jeffrey Hopkins, from* The Tantric Distinction

POWER OF POSITIVITY

My name is Thubten Lodrö. I am a Tibetan Buddhist monk, twenty-seven years old, born in France. I introduce myself in this way only to talk about a lama, Thubten Shenphen Rinpoche, with whom I have had the great opportunity to stand behind.

Shenphen Rinpoche grew up in France, too, and when he was sixteen years old, he entered Nalanda Monastery in France, where he took first monk vows with Geshe Jampa Tegchok (who later become Abbot of Sera-Jhe Monastery in south India). He was recognized later on as the incarnation of Lama Gendune Rabgye and in 1990 he took full ordination with His Holiness the Dalai Lama. During his first "monk years," he set up his first nonprofit organization and made numerous humanitarian trips to India, where he built a little dispensary, gave healings, and built showers for people. He set up a sponsoring system for Tibetan refugees and programs in France to help children and adults with social, moral, and educational needs.

I would like to tell you about a young child named Toni, whom Shenphen Rinpoche helped. He was from Russia and was very sick, having been stricken with a rare, treatment-resistant form of leukemia.

Lama Shenphen heard about this child via the Internet, when someone asked him to pray for him, as he is known to be a healer. Lama engaged himself immediately and made plans to go see Toni in Germany, where he was living with his mother. After a few days, Lama decided to reorganize his schedule and radically changed his center on the island of Paros in Greece where he was living in order to welcome the child and give him a calmer environment for healing. All the dharma students there were very moved by how Lama-la was taking care of this child, and how that child was considering him as his father. He raised funds for the child and immediately asked for prayers and pujas around the world.

Toni was a very sensitive child, but he was also very nervous and hyperactive, close to being aggressive. Being with him was not easy because he could take all your time, attention, and energy. But it was amazing how soon after being with Lama

Shenphen that Toni became quieter and less anxious. He began thinking about how to help those around him. Even though Toni was only nine years old, he understood that the monk he considered as his father, his best friend, and his teacher would remain close to him, no matter what happened to him.

When a relapse was diagnosed, Lama-la went with Toni to Berlin and spent seven days and six nights a week with him, living in the hospital. At each operation Toni had to go through, Lama Shenphen stayed close to him—when they gave him anesthesia, and again when he was waking up. Toni decided to become Buddhist, and he was given the name "Thubten Norbu," but we all called him "Toni-Norbu" [Norbu means "Precious Gem"]. Inspired by the love and care Lama Shenphen showed him, he also wanted to become a monk and began asking for teachings from his hospital bed in order to teach and help others later on. Nine months after he met Lama Shenphen, Toni-Norbu passed away, with "his Lama" at his side.

Those of us who were involved will never forget Toni, who was truly an exceptional child. For me the most moving part of this story was to see how one person with the right attitude at the right moment could inspire so much positivity in others—through prayer, discussions, and self-engagement—and thus change the minds of so many. That was especially true of this young child, who despite his own illness and suffering, was praying for the other sick children in the hospital at the time he was dying. It makes me deeply feel and appreciate how vast the mind truly is and how precious all those beings are who are here only to benefit others.

—*Ven. Thubten Lodrö*

> When we see somebody who is very sick and in terrible pain, even though we see only a single person who is going through this experience, we can learn to see that person as a representative of the entirety of sentient beings who are undergoing the same kind of torture at that very moment.
>
> —*Geshe Tsultrim Gyeltsen*

WAKEUP CALL

During the years I lived with Nyoshul Khenpo Rinpoche and served as his attendant, I was with him almost every day. Once I remember when he and Tulku Pema Wangyal had just returned from a trip to Bordeaux or perhaps Brittany, along France's southern Atlantic shore, where they had given some teachings. In Tibet and throughout the Himalayas, people have no beach to go to, and certainly monks in some traditions are prohibited from swimming. So it must have been the first time Khenpo had seen the beach and observed exactly what Westerners do there. When he came back to the monastery, he began to give us dharma teachings about the eight worldly pitfalls—pleasure and pain, loss and gain, fame and shame, praise and blame—and then suddenly started talking about the beach and how he and Tulku had gone to the very edge of the ocean.

"It was so *big,*" he said in almost childlike awe, calling it something like King Trident's House, "thc house of the king of the ocean." And then he excitedly described what he had seen. "There were these people there, and instead of sitting and meditating or doing yoga, these people were just lying there—almost naked!—and doing nothing! And when they were tired of lying there, instead of doing something they just turned over! And then they lay there again for another few hours!"

Khenpo was truly, genuinely, perplexed. In retrospect, he almost sounded as if he were out of *Third Rock from the Sun,* the TV show about aliens coming down to earth. "Why were they doing that?" he asked over and over. Though he couldn't understand it, he had so much compassion for them. "How could they waste their precious human existence?" he continued. "This life that is so short, so tenuous, so precious, so valuable, so *necessary,* a life not to be squandered but to be used impeccably and usefully for the benefit and welfare of all—a life to be used to think about the future in the next life, not just to lounge around all day in the hot sun like a big sleeping lizard!" Khenpo was sincerely impassioned now. "I just wanted to go wake them up!"

Then he had noticed there was a big white chair about fifty meters away—obviously the lifeguard's post. "But there were two young people sitting there," he said, "so I couldn't go up there. But I wanted to badly, because I wanted to climb up there and announce to everybody it was time to wake up!"

For all of us Westerners who heard Khenpo's live report from the beach that day, we realized how truly empty our habits of indulgence were in the face of such devotion to life.

—Lama Surya Das

Generosity . . . arises when the Bodhisattva is intoxicated by compassion and is no longer aware of himself. His mind is not merely filled with compassion, it becomes compassion, it is COMPASSION.

—*Chögyam Trungpa Rinpoche*

COMPASSIONATE EATING

When I was a small child in Tibet, I saw some people slaughtering animals for food—goats and sheep—and it upset me so much I started to cry. I even had to look away. So at a very early age I began to think about the suffering of beings, not just in the human realm and all the different kinds of suffering there, but in all the hell realms too. Everywhere. And I began to see how all beings, without exception, are caught up in the ultimate suffering of samsara, that is to say, cyclic existence. It's very important to actually feel that suffering in your own being, to take time and contemplate it. Then it becomes real.

For example, if you eat meat, then it's very important to think about the suffering those animals went through and try to actually really feel it yourself. And if you eat meat, then you should say prayers and many mantras for the benefit of these very beings you are eating so that they might be free of their suffering in the next life. You can even go to a place where animals are slaughtered and say prayers for them. And then having done this for those beings who gave their life for your pleasure, you can begin to do this for all beings, so that you come to feel that their suffering is not separate from you, that their suffering *is* your suffering. To understand how to be kind to others, you really have to understand the nature of suffering. And it is out of this kind of understanding that real kindness can arise.

—*Penor Rinpoche*

> Enlightenment will be ours when we are able to care for others as much as we now care for ourselves.
>
> —*Dilgo Khyentse Rinpoche*

THE EQUALITY OF ALL THAT LIVES

In 1982 His Holiness the Dalai Lama of Tibet was dining in France with Pawo Rinpoche X. The pair was recounting stories of the past and anticipating the rebirth of the recently deceased Gyalwa Karmapa.

Just then the elderly Pawo Rinpoche spied an ant struggling across the polished floor, wending its way toward the sun.

The aged Pawo Rinpoche no longer had the use of his legs. He requested the Dalai Lama to be so kind as to rescue the little creature and help it on its way.

His Holiness did so with alacrity, blessing the insect with a whispered benediction. Gently, he carried the insect across the regal chamber and set it down safely in the warm sun. Chuckling with delight, he rejoined his venerable colleague.

"Now I have done a service for you, Rinpoche. Your old eyes are better than mine! People talk about emptiness . . . but loving regard for the equality of all that lives is the true sign of a bodhisattva."

His Holiness later recounted the story, during a teaching in France about the necessity for compassion, selfless service, and universal responsibility.

"My religion is kindness," he stated.

—*Lama Surya Das,*

from The Snow Lion's Turquoise Mane

BODHI RISING

On a recent trip to Japan on a spiritual pilgrimage, I was staying in a hotel in the sea city of Atami, with a balcony overlooking the great Pacific Ocean. Yukiko, my roommate, was a Japanese-born woman who moved me deeply with her quiet presence and inner strength, for she had battled a catastrophic illness and survived. For the first two nights, we had been simply too tired to pull ourselves out of bed to see the legendary sunrise over Atami's waters, but on our last morning I was determined to share the beauty of it with her. Just as the lush red dome was peeping over the horizon, I ran to the cold balcony in bare feet, calling out to Yukiko to follow. Each second this great eastern ball of fire rose higher and higher, fabulous in color and size, but Yukiko was nowhere to be found. I became so irritated she was missing the view. Where *was* she? Then suddenly, seconds too late, she arrived at my shoulder looking a bit sheepish—holding out slippers and a heavier kimono for me. My heart broke. While I had been thinking only about the sunrise, she had been thinking only of my comfort.

—*Pamela Bloom*

PLANTING MERIT

We raised many cows at Sosa Monastery. Sometimes they gave birth to stillborn calves. Whenever that happened, somehow the people from our town or the next town knew it right away and came to ask for the meat. Since our diet was purely vegetarian, and since the calf must have been born at our monastery due to a close karmic tie with us, we couldn't imagine eating the meat.

When we gave away the stillborn calf while wishing, "Feed those people with your flesh; and may you plant as much merit as you can," people took it gratefully. But sometimes no one would come to claim the meat. Usually people came within two hours of the birth to take the meat, but once in a while no one came even after a full day.

Our master said that if the calf had planted merit in its past incarnations, people would come to take the meat, and the calf would accumulate more merit. But if the calf had not planted any merit, people would not come, and there would be no one to help the calf plant any merit. He said that when a cow is killed in a slaughterhouse and becomes food for thousands of people, it plants the merit of feeding others with its flesh. If it is reincarnated as a human, it become a wealthy person, with between two hundred and one thousand bags of rice a year.

Master Baek meant that when you feed others with your own flesh, you accumulate great merit.

Once no one asked for the merit of one stillborn calf, and eventually the meat went bad. When the master saw that, he told us to bury the carcass and plant a fruit tree over it. If you feed ripened fruit that has used a calf as fertilizer to spiritual seekers, the calf gets to plant merit. However, it was during the summer, and I couldn't get a fruit tree, nor was there anyone around who knew about fruit trees, so I was at a loss. I had to at least plant a willow tree. After four years, the willow grew large, fed by the nutrients of the calf's carcass.

That winter, we had other firewood, but I intentionally used the wood from the willow tree and heated the rooms of many spiritual seekers. As I was heating the rooms, I invoked a wŏn [a prayer] to Buddha, "By the merit of keeping these spiritual seekers warm, may this calf meet enlightened masters, listen to their teachings and awaken to their teachings in every future incarnation, so that he may serve and accumulate great merit before Buddha. . . !" Until I had done that, it had been a burden in my mind, but when I used the firewood and made the wŏn, I felt as if a weight had been lifted from my shoulders. I realize that my master had given me the task to make me practice compassion.

After that incident, even when a monastery's cat dies, we buried it with a thoughtful wŏn. We always found something that might accumulate merit for the past owner of its body.

—*Master Jae Woong Kim,*
from Polishing the Diamond, Enlightening the Mind

SACRED CRITICISM

I began my writing career as a music critic. I love music and it was a great privilege to interview famous musicians and attend their concerts. I have to admit there was also a very real thrill of seeing my name in print. Though I had had little personal experience in rock and roll, I had been trained as a musician and this knowledge combined with some writing skill helped propel me up the ladder from one prestigious magazine and newspaper to another. As with many critics, it was easy to get lost in the power of the position. Though it is not always the case, the role of critic can be a vehicle for all sorts of petty opinions and unresolved anger, a license to vent. I tried not to misuse the position but at times I did write a number of "bad" reviews. All the way, I tried to distance myself from the person I was writing about.

Then one day a famous musician wrote a letter to my publication condemning the review I had written about his latest recording, and, to my horror, the publication printed it. His attack was quite personal—understandably so—but it really hurt, and I experienced the sting of being shamed in public. From that moment on, the joy of reviewing music quickly began to diminish, for I had had more than a glimpse of the pain I had possibly been causing others through my career. Day after day, I asked myself, how can this type of writing become of benefit to others? Not just to the reader, but to the performer him or herself? There weren't any easy answers.

Then one day I had the chance to review a very unusual cabaret singer, an older actress who was very soulful but also very eccentric. Her untrained singing voice, however, was in a million pieces and some of her "characters" were not yet "there." But as I sat down to write the review, a mere three hundred words, something took me over and suddenly I had a vision of what this performer could truly be in her highest form. And that's the review I wrote, not really of the performance I saw but a description of her soul. After the review was published, the performer hunted me down to say she had been floored by what I had written. No one, she said, had *ever* seen her this way, and it was exactly how she saw herself at her most ideal. It was like a blueprint, she said, for her future work. But most of all, the review had given her, she said, the hope to persevere in her soul's work. Hearing her happiness filled my heart. That was ten or fifteen years ago, and today I am thrilled to see she is still performing. And a recent review I read of her work shows she has truly mastered that ideal.

As I write this, I remember the moment when I first met His Holiness Gyalwa Karmapa, the head of the Kagyu lineage of Tibetan Buddhism, in the early eighties. I had been practicing sitting meditation for a few years, but I found it simply excruciating. In a small group interview with this great meditation master, I somehow had the courage to drop all pretense and complain.

"I just hate sitting practice," I remember saying. "It's excruciating. I'm so antsy. I can't sit still. I bother everybody around me by moving around. Deep inside me I feel how important it is, but still—I hate it. I don't know what to do."

His Holiness just looked at me for a long time, as if seeing very deeply into me. I thought perhaps he was trying to figure out how to criticize me or put me in my place, but then he took a deep breath and said very, very slowly, "I think—if you continue to practice—in ten or fifteen years—it is—going to get—*easier.*"

I was stunned. I almost thought he was joking. But he was perfectly serious. And he was right. It did get easier. After ten or fifteen years. But if he hadn't said it to me then, I don't think I would have ever had the courage and the motivation to continue. In that moment, quite subtly he gave me the sacred vision to persevere.

How often we think that the only way to improve upon that which needs growth is to criticize. Together, both experiences taught me that sacred vision is more powerful than criticism, and that compassion is the elixir of life.

—*Pamela Bloom*

BEYOND PROTEST

In the sixties I spent a lot of time working with human rights. In the early years, I was sometimes more motivated by fear and saw some of the painful results of that ego at work. I remember a sit-in at a small Southern lunch counter. We were two Northern students, so young and so self-righteous. We had no idea what those in the town were thinking and feeling, and we did not want to know. We only wanted to express our viewpoint and righteousness. We wanted to change them.

We came into the lunchroom and sat at the counter, facing the glares of those sitting around us. The cook just looked at us and asked what we wanted. "Coke, milkshake, doughnut" came our replies. We were feeling smug; was it really this easy? He gathered some items and carried them to the counter. I remember how he approached me with my doughnut and the large glass of Coke, sweat-covered from its icy contents. I looked at the glass with pleasure since the day was hot. He reached out with the glass, and with no hesitation poured it over my head. While I sat there in shock, he crumbled the doughnut over me too. The second counterman did the same to my partner. Then he nodded, and others at the counter simply picked us up, two young women, one white and one black, carried us out the door, dumped us on the curb, and locked the door behind us.

In those early days, I totally lacked compassion for this opposition. They were wrong and I was right; it was that simple. I had no ability to be present with their pain nor to hear them. I had no ability to be present with my own fear nor hear myself.

Years passed and I did learn. It was a tough learning, a fruit of many tears and bruises, of much pain and confusion. But slowly, I did learn the power of compassion and presence. No one incident was my primary teacher, but I do remember a few hours in a small jail. One of my cell partners was an older, Southern black woman, large of body and with soft, deep eyes. She wore a black dress covered with red roses and a tiny hat still adorned her head. I was angry at what had happened that particular day, an incident not too different from the one above. I was expressing that anger, muttering, pacing the cell. After about an hour she walked up to me so sweetly and in a kind voice invited me to sit down. "Aren't you angry too?" I asked her. "Yes," she replied, "but I also love them, sweetheart, and they are so afraid." She hugged me gently as I wept. She taught me with those simple words that anger and compassion were not mutually exclusive. It was the first time my eyes really opened to what was happening around me, and from this sister, whose name I never even knew, I began to learn the power of love.

—*Barbara Brodsky*

FINAL GIFTS

Jetsunma Ahkön Norbu Lhamo, an American tulku of Jewish-Italian background, belongs to the Nyingma tradition of Tibetan Buddhism. She was recognized as the reincarnation of the seventeenth-century founder of the Palyul lineage and monastery by Padma Norbu (Penor) Rinpoche in 1987 and formerly enthroned in 1988. She is the resident teacher of Kunzang Palyul Chöling in Poolesville, Maryland.

The day my eldest daughter graduated from high school was also the day that one of my oldest friends in the dharma began his transition from this life. That day is one of the most intensely memorable days I have ever experienced. It taught me about transitions in all aspects of my life and gave me an incredible glimpse into the compassionate nature of my teacher.

Early that day our teacher Jetsunma Akhön Lhamo called about two dozen of her students together to be at the bedside of our friend because she knew his time was at hand. She invited us to do round-the-clock prayers for his benefit. It was the first time that we were present at the death of one of our own since we became a community nearly twenty years earlier, even though Jetsunma herself had assisted at this most important transition on numerous occasions.

In terrible pain and overwhelmed by fear, our friend was slowly making his exit. At his side were his two sons, both attending to his physical needs. Our friend took comfort in the presence of his sons, but his attention was riveted upon his teacher. It was clear that he knew she was the doorway to everything at that moment. Several years earlier he had left our community to go off on his own, but when diagnosed with cancer came back to practice. Jetsunma welcomed him with open arms, much like the father in the famous story of the prodigal son.

Here our friend now lay, with complete confidence that his teacher would be there for him. And indeed she was. Jetsunma never once left his side during the thirty-six hours that we were together, even though most of us got up and took a break.

Jetsunma was there like a mother for her only son. She had a power about her I had not experienced before. Her energy was anchored, focused, unshakable, present, intense like a thunderclap and far-reaching like a vortex that extended far into space. She seemed aware of every nuance of my friend's physical and spiritual situation. She advised him, reassured him, gently shifted his focus away from his pain, and suggested how the attending nurses might make him more comfortable. Periodically she touched the top of his head.

Shortly before his transition, she invited us to feel his fontanel. I was amazed at how open it was. . . . It was soft like a baby's and protruding out. I knew that this opening was a miraculous display of our teacher's compassionate activity. With our hearts at our knees, we were grateful that now he would be able to move his consciousness out through the top of his head at the time of his death, assuring him an auspicious rebirth. In that moment, I was overcome with emotion. I understood the preciousness of having a root guru.

—*Sylvia Somerville*

> There is no greater act of charity you can give than helping a person to die well.
>
> —*Sogyal Rinpoche*

LAUGHING HEART

Some of the most moving acts of compassion I have ever seen have been among some of the poorest people on earth. The Zangskar Valley of Ladakh is situated in a remote corner of the Indian Himalayas. The people eke out their living from high altitude desert soil that is under snow for nine months of the year. To help some of the women get an education, I often travel to this pristine yet desolate region, even when it means trekking for days over mountains, avalanches, and treacherous waters. Invariably I am met with extraordinary kindness wherever I go.

Although the people of Zangskar are ethnically Tibetan, due to the vagaries of history, they now live in a Muslim district of a disputed territory in northern India, struggling for physical, political, and cultural survival. Without adequate schools, medical care, or nutrition, their only comfort is the Buddhist faith of their ancestors and their love and devotion for the Dalai Lama.

One summer, as soon as the snows had melted, I journeyed to the region with a Zangskari nun friend. Descending from the icy mountain pass, we stopped at the house of an aunt. The woman had recently lost her husband to an avalanche and each of her children had only a single shirt to wear, despite the bitter cold. Yet despite her empty larder, the aunt poured us endless cups of butter tea in her mud-floored, smoke-filled kitchen. A huge, genuine smile came with every cup as she compassionately anticipated every need.

The love of family and friends was the family's only wealth, but it was immense. Laughter was their gift to one another.

Such generosity of spirit in the midst of astonishing poverty can only come from a heart of pure love, teaching all of us life's greatest meaning.

—*Karma Lekshe Tsomo*

PERFECT STRANGER

I live in New York City, and I am the kind of person who doesn't like to make too much contact with people on the street. Maybe it's a form of neurotic protection, maybe it's a little reasonable. One day, crazy with deadlines, I was rushing to pack for an overseas trip, make a doctor's appointment, and get my taxes to my accountant on time. With eight minutes to get to FedEx, I hurried out of the coffee shop where I'd eaten. Halfway down the block, I realized I was going in the wrong direction and turned around abruptly—at which point, a pedestrian right behind ran into me. To my mind, it was so slight a bump it could have gone unnoticed. But this other man who ran into me started yelling: "How can you be so stupid?! You haven't been aware since the moment you left that coffee shop. You just can't go bumping into people right and left." His tone was really derisive. For some reason he had been nipping at my heels for more than a block.

I was outraged. My knee-jerk reaction was to say, "You * * *, it's a free sidewalk. If you hadn't been walking so close to me, this never would have happened." In fact I did say a little of that (without the cursing), which of course only got him madder. He let out a new torrent of invectives. But as I watched him become apoplectic, something happened. All the teachings I had been studying about compassion came back to me and it was as if something in me shifted. In that moment, I genuinely felt that this man was suffering as much, if not more, than me. I didn't want his day, or mine, ruined. So I yelled out, "Excuse me," hoping to say something nice, but he started walking away, yelling over his back, "Don't even *try*. . ." and kept walking. At which point I did something I could never have imagined myself doing. I ran to catch up with him, put my hand very gently but firmly on his arm, and waited until we had made complete eye contact. Then I said very, very slowly, with utter genuineness, "I'm sorry. I'm *really* sorry."

He was speechless. I don't think he had ever received a response to his anger like that. And I had never been so intimate with a stranger. Time stopped for both of us and for a split second

I think both of us saw the other as a real person. Then he sputtered, "Well . . . uh . . . yeah . . . well . . . I guess you had a lot on your mind." He then whipped around and walked away fast.

I watched his figure receding in the wash of the street lamp and my heart filled . . . with what? Dare I say, *love?* At the very least, a deep gratefulness. Here was a perfect stranger pointing out the chaos of my mind, showing me how even a moment of mindlessness can cause suffering, and then inspiring me to make a leap over years of self-imposed limitations.

New York!

—*Pamela Bloom*

EXTRAORDINARY CROSSINGS

I was born near Lhasa on a farm, and at about one year of age I was recognized as the reincarnation of a long line of Tarab Tulkus and taken to the Tashi Rabten Monastery in Kongpo in the southeast of Tibet. The Tarab lamas had long been the spiritual leaders of the Tashi Rabten area, which was about two thousand square kilometers, including a monastery and large *lhadrang,* or estate, that the Tarab lamas had inherited from their former predecessors. Upon my entrance into Drepung Monastery University in Lhasa, I had the spiritual duty, as a lama with a large estate, to make offerings (money, food, and tea) to all the monks and to give special gifts to the teachers, abbots, and officials of Drepung. Such it was that I found myself at the age of six accompanied by a huge party as I traveled from Kongpo to Lhasa to begin my studies. With us were numerous representatives from my monastery, my estate, and from the surrounding area itself. Also, we had about forty mules carrying all the offerings, including Tibetan tea for 10,000 monks. So we were a huge caravan—mules, horses, people—traveling together for about three weeks along rigorous paths. Nowadays it takes perhaps only about four hours by car to get to Lhasa from there.

When we were about three days from Lhasa, we had to cross the great Lhasa River. At that time there was no bridge, though later the Chinese would build one over Lhasa River, much closer to the city. I remember it was the ninth month of the Tibetan calendar year 1941 in the late autumn or beginning of winter. Already a lot of ice was flowing in the river and we were all standing on the bank looking at these thick ice flakes. After a time people started to panic because if we did not cross at that moment, we would not be able to reach the place before sunset where the horses and mules could find grass to eat for the night. But we did not know how long it would take for the ice to flow by.

The pieces of ice were quite big—about one meter across and thick. So not knowing what else to do, my manager and my teacher came to me and said, "You are the lama, so now you have to do something to help us to go across." So I asked, "Why could we not just go across?" They explained that the ice was very heavy and coming with a great force with the water, and if the horses and mules were to step into the water, the ice would break their legs. So there was no way we could cross under these bad conditions. And if we did not manage to cross very soon, the animals would have no food for the night.

On hearing this, I prayed for the animals and a great feeling of love and compassion for them arose. Everybody was standing there at the riverbank gazing at the water and the ice while I was praying. Not more than five minutes had lapsed when the impossible happened. Just at the place where we had to cross, the water suddenly became free of ice, the large pieces staying back and piling up as if someone were actually holding them back, even though the water was still flowing. Immediately all sixty horses and mules crossed, and as soon as the last animal jumped up onto the riverbank on the other side, the ice started to float quickly down the river again.

We were all quite shocked and rather speechless, but at that moment I was so happy, not only for the horses and men, but because I had had the experience of compassion, faith, and prayer in one. After that, there was no doubt in peoples' minds that I was a true reincarnation.

—*Tarab Tulku XI*

HIGHER LOVE

When Ivan and Teresa Milton came together some twenty years ago, both knew Ivan had a deep yearning to become a Buddhist monk. But at that time they were both madly in love and determined to get married. So Ivan's desire to become a monk was left to the future. Over the years, their ongoing interest in Buddhism and work as psychotherapists in Melbourne, Australia, brought them into contact with many Buddhist teachers.

I met them four years ago and was immediately struck by their empathy with the suffering beings of this world. Although these two people had met every material need in their lives, they nevertheless felt they had to listen to their deep spiritual yearnings. Though their marriage and psychotherapy work proved to be a source of growth for both of them, Ivan's wish to become a monk had not gone away.

Teresa supported Ivan's long-held wish. If Ivan were to become a monk, she decided, she could happily live as his ex-wife who had consented to his ordination and would not feel as if he had spurned her. She even promised to support him if it became necessary.

Her love for Ivan in no way meant possessing him but rather letting him aspire to what might benefit him most, thus deepening her own loving-kindness. This process of mutual letting go was accompanied by ever-increasing feelings of kindness between the two, and in these feelings Ivan realized why he had married Teresa so many years before. Their mutual devotion to care for each other had a unique loving quality that attracted all beings close to their hearts.

A year after their seeking my advice at the Atisha Centre in Melbourne, Ivan was ordained as a Buddhist monk by His Eminence Chogye Trichen Rinpoche. In the same week, Teresa took celibate vows with Lama Zopa Rinpoche in Melbourne.

Before Ivan's departure for Nepal to be ordained, they conducted a touching ceremony at Melbourne Airport. Teresa described it to me in an e-mail: "We had a little ceremony at the airport, just before the final gate of parting (literal and metaphorical). We took off our wedding rings, I returned mine to Ivan and he returned his to me, and then we placed them in the little box (in which we originally bought them for our wedding) as an offering to His Eminence and all Holy Beings for the sake of all creatures. We both cried from sadness and inexplicable joy, and some profound unlabeled feelings. The dissolution ceremony had much more impact on us than the wedding ceremony."

As Ivan and Teresa dissolved their worldly marriage, tears of joy in their spiritual bond welled in their eyes.

In a card Ivan presented to Teresa just before his departure, he wrote: "If only everyone could share what we have found with and through each other. That should be our wish. That this sublime emergence will spread beyond you and me and into the hearts of everyone we meet. May they all be touched by this love."

After the ordination ceremony in Nepal, His Eminence Chogye Trichen Rinpoche told Ivan that the wedding rings would be melted down and applied to an altar image or a thangka. Not many wedding rings see their next incarnation as ornamentation on a sacred image! And I am certain that their tears contained no elements of sadness or loss but only of joy and happiness, which their many friends continue to share.

The occasion of a person taking ordination can sometimes be accompanied by feelings of sadness and rejection. To the contrary, Ivan's ordination and Teresa's vow of celibacy have given so many of their friends reasons to rejoice in a profound life change that has been achieved without any great difficulty. For them it has manifested as happiness deriving from mutual acceptance and the maturity of a relationship that surely must have begun many lifetimes before.

—*Lama Choedak Yuthok*

SACRED FOOD

It was a good time in my life, professionally and personally, yet I was inordinately tired. This led me to consult with a Chinese acupuncturist. He treated me and suggested that I see him weekly. During one of our subsequent sessions, he advised me I needed to eat salmon. As a committed vegetarian for almost twenty years, these words flowed right through me and I ignored them. Over the next six to twelve months, he brought up this issue with increasing regularity. After awhile I could not ignore him. The acupuncture treatments were helping, but I knew I was not yet well and had to do something about it. I finally bought a piece of salmon, brought it home, and it rotted in the refrigerator. This reoccurred several times over the next few months. All the while pressure from the doctor was mounting. Again, I went to the store, forced myself to buy yet another piece of salmon, cooked it three days later, but ended up giving it to the animals outside. My whole being was screaming "NO!" But as time went on, neither the acupuncturist nor the weakness in my body would let me forget that I was ill. Finally I went to the store again, bought some salmon, brought it home, and cooked it. As I sat at the table with this once living being whose life had been taken, not given, I was face to face with one of the biggest moral and ethical dilemmas of my life. I wanted to heal, but I didn't want my healing to be contingent on the death of another. When I finally forced myself to take my first bite, I felt my heart completely break. How would I ever be able to reconcile these seemingly incompatible truths? But as I continued this excruciating process, I was surprised to find that over time I became very close to salmon. I started to feel the medicine in the salmon and my gratitude for what it was giving me became enormous.

Then my doctor told me I needed to eat chicken, and then eventually red meat. I remember the first time I ate red meat, during a meditation weekend after the doctor had insisted I add meat to my diet. I was sitting in a fellow meditator's house, hanging out on the sofa at break time with other people. On the plate before me was this piece of meat and I remember sitting and sobbing my eyes out because I simply did not know how to be in right relationship with this animal who had given its life so that I might live. That was when I really got it—that it had given its *life* to me—and it just deepened my gratitude profoundly. Once I realized my closeness to this being, to all beings, then I could partake of their offering. It was at that moment that the act of eating meat became a sacred relationship. And it was the beginning of my healing.

—*P'nina Macher*

Buddhists believe that whatever we do in this life will plant karmic seeds that will result in our next birth and its conditions. Consequently, we should be careful of our actions of body, speech, and mind. If we know that at each moment we are creating something for the future, we should be happy. We have the opportunity to make our actions good so that the consequences will be good for us and for others. If we strive at every moment to work selflessly for the good of all beings, then we can truly speak of a new life at every moment.

—*Master Sheng-yen*

THE MUSIC OF LETTING GO

Before I started to meditate, my work as a jazz pianist was motivated a lot by ego. What was most important to me back then was competition, fame, getting reviewed, and getting ahead in the business, which is all driven by a basic lack of self-esteem, a lack of belief in oneself. But the more I continued on my musical path, the more people I met who drew me in the opposite direction—in particular, a saxophonist named Bill Harper who was very much into Sufism and was able to combine his wonderful sense of music with his spiritual practice. I worked with his band for about four years. Then I went through a number of transitions. I got married, my father died, I got my first house, I had a serious accident that affected my hands, I got divorced—all within a space of two or three years. It was a very dark period with a lot of anger and sadness, but I had been practicing yoga for three or four years before that, so I relied on my spiritual practice at that point to carry me through. Perhaps it was because of the pain, but through those experiences something inside me got loosened and fell away. I started playing music from a totally different point of view. Shortly after that I moved to New Jersey and joined a sangha group that started out as a kripalu yoga support group. The leader changed it into a Vipassana meditation group and everyone dropped out except me and the leader. Since then, the sangha has grown to about sixty people meditating together on a weekly basis and attending retreats. It has been a wonderful opportunity for me to not only do the practice but also establish friendships and a new community revolving around spiritual practice.

I discovered through Vipassana meditation that compassion begins with oneself. In the midst of this terrible time, I realized there was something there that I wasn't seeing and that was the witness inside me. It felt revolutionary to realize that I am not my anger, not my depression, not my sadness; these are just mind-states that come and go. Slowly I began to understand that other people are going through their difficulties too, and that suffering is universal, that my suffering is everybody's suffering. One of the turning points came when I read that if you can't feel compassion for yourself, just try being compassionate toward someone else and that will help you be compassionate toward yourself. So I said okay, I can try that. I may not be able to fully feel compassion for myself, but if I can do it for someone else, then I will just practice that. That's where I am right now.

As I practiced Vipassana meditation, I found there was less a sense of feeling driven and therefore more a sense of relaxation in my music. I became more comfortable with slower tempos, gentler harmonies. For a while I was writing music with a lot of dissonance, a lot of anger, a lot of complexity and darkness, but meditation practice helped my music become lighter, harmonically speaking, and I think it also affected my technique. At some point I made a very conscious decision that I wanted to play music for people to listen to and enjoy, and not just for myself, or my friends in the group, or for a specific audience in the music business. I felt that if I can't play music that someone totally unschooled can sit down and enjoy, then I am not really doing what I am supposed to be doing, which is to benefit others to the best of my ability.

The solo CD I just finished was totally improvised. On the night of a full moon I just turned on the recording equipment I had set up in my house and started to play—one piece after another. I could never have planned that in a million years, but it was perfect just as it was. Months later, when I listened to the music for the first time, I thought, something happened in this album for which I was not responsible. Something just came through me and sang.

—*Armen Donelian*

In general, we feel that the result of any activity we do, whether it is artistic or otherwise, depends upon the goodness of mind. And therefore, any music or artistic form, if it is performed with a view of aggrandizing one's self, removing one's own immediate discomfort, gaining profit or fame, or drawing attention to one's self in any way, will not be good. But if it is done with forgetting one's self and only concerned with how to be of benefit to others, to inspire them, to cheer them, wishing them well and to be free of disturbances rather than further heightening their negative afflictions, then it is almost certain that one's creations would be excellent.

—*Venerable Lungri Namgyal*

MEDICINE BUDDHA

The former physician to His Holiness Dalai Lama, Dr. Yeshi Dhonden is one of the foremost Tibetan doctors of the world. We met in the United States. A year and a half after witnessing his great diagnostic skills both on rounds and at various clinics, including my office in Massachusetts, I decided to go to India at his invitation. In the spring of 1983, just as I was arriving exhausted after a thirty-six-hour journey, he announced that we were leaving the very next day to go to Bombay. Dr. Dhonden is very well known and highly respected in India, and as a result hundreds of people come to see him at one time. During the next two weeks, we saw 1,096 patients.

My job during this visit was to do triage—to manage the patients coming in and out of the office—but at some point there was just no more room and it seemed humanly impossible to see one more patient. One day there was a knock on the door. Standing there was a very forlorn-looking man, slumped over and exhausted, holding in his arms his frail, pale eleven-year-old daughter. With tears in his eyes he told me she had leukemia and that it had taken them days to travel there. Apparently the outside office had already informed him that there was no possible way for Dr. Dhonden to see them, but he wouldn't give up. "Couldn't you please find room for her to be seen?" he begged. I didn't know what to say. We were so overwhelmed, there were so many people sitting in the hospital waiting room without appointments, and in the office with Dr. Dhonden there were always two or three patients waiting. I looked at him and said, "I am really sorry, I just don't see how we can fit one more person into the schedule because we are already seeing ten times more than we planned on." At that moment, Dr. Dhonden, who obviously was very busy with other patients and doesn't even speak English, somehow understood what I was saying and beckoned to me from across the room to let the man in. I was stunned but I did it, and he never mentioned the incident.

Later, somebody approached me to invite Dr. Dhonden, his pharmacist, his translator, and myself to their home for dinner. This often happens when Dr. Dhonden travels in India because it is considered a great honor, like a blessing, to have him in one's home. I checked with Dr. Dhonden and he said yes, so that evening we went to this house. To my shock, when we arrived, we found thirteen people sitting in the living room waiting to see Dr. Dhonden as patients. It was at the end of the day and Dr. Dhonden had not stopped working for one minute. I became very upset and said to the host, "How could you do such a thing? Dr. Dhonden has been working so hard, you invited us to dinner, and you have all these patients to be seen." Then I went into the bedroom and started to cry. Right there and then, Dr. Dhonden came in after me and said very strongly: "How could you be so upset and angry with them? You can't do that. They are patients. They come for my help. A doctor has a responsibility to help a patient when they are asked." And then he left me to return to them. After composing myself, I followed. He saw all the patients first and then we had dinner.

Although I had witnessed Dr. Dhonden with hundreds of patients in the U.S, there was no comparison to this introduction to Tibetan clinics in India. Indeed, that visit began chiseling and reshaping my own definition and understanding of what it means to practice love and compassion, essentials for being a good doctor. All my life I've been a helper and I have always gone the extra mile, but Dr. Dhonden showed me what the real stretch is. Through his untiring example over the last nineteen years, he has shown me again and again how to go the one-millionth mile.

—Marsha Woolf

> Because their value is equal, many pieces of gold are worth more than a single coin. So it is with sentient beings—many are more precious than one. Fortified with that awareness, one can live and act accordingly—with simplicity, generosity, and respect for life. The attitude of cherishing all sentient beings as though they were truly the same as you is a deeply moving and personal experience. It is a life-changer. It is also the cause of happiness.
>
> *—Jetsunma Akhön Norbu Lhamo*

HEALING BODY AND SOUL

When I began to get rheumatoid arthritis, I was in my seventh year of Zen practice. In just a few months, my hands, feet, hips, and knees became totally crippled. I simply couldn't get out of bed. Thank God I was living in a Zen community where people took care of me. But I was very wary of men. When I was growing up, my dad had an explosive temper and seeing my mom appease him for many years I vowed I would never marry. I felt like I would never ever put myself in situations where I was dependent on someone who might hurt me. Though I was attracted to men, I came to abhor my own sex drive and saw men as only interested in me as an object of desire.

But when I got sick, the first thing that happened was that a man in the community, a Zen priest, started coming over to my apartment where I lived with other Zen students. He would say, "Oh, I don't have any food in my office," and then pour himself a bowl of cereal. All the while, he would be checking out the cupboards and then would go shopping and bring food over. One day when I was lying in bed and didn't care whether I lived or died, he came over and said he was taking me to a place where I could heal. Over my weak protests, he picked me up, threw some underwear into a paperbag, then drove me out to the ocean where his girlfriend had a house. From their porch and living room window you could look out on the waves and the garden. I spent a couple of weeks there. That was the beginning of gaining the little energy I needed to think about the rest of my life. During this time he even took my young son, who was close in age to his son, to Texas to visit Indian reservations.

Also, during this same time, my ex-boyfriend, the father of my child, would come to my apartment regularly with other Zen students and drive me around the mountains to soak in the beauty of nature. One time they even found a wheelchair, piled me into the car, and took me to an art gallery where they wheeled me around. It was absolutely fabulous, after lying in bed day after day looking only at the design on the sheets and the paint chipped on the window sill, to see these vibrant wonderful paintings.

Later, when I was starting to walk again, my brother and dad came to see me. I hadn't told them about the illness because I never wanted to expose my vulnerable side to my father. When my dad saw me, he immediately said he was taking me to Acapulco to be restored by the sun and warm water. He even gave me few hundred dollars for a new wardrobe. I couldn't get out of my lounge chair, but my dad helped me up and down the ladder in the pool. This was the beginning of a very good therapy for me.

At the end of this long period, when I finally began to work again, I saw that I no longer thought about men in the same way. All these men had come out of the woodwork to help and support me without any thought of sex. I know that is a funny thing to say, but it is the first time I saw men as human beings. Women helped me too, bathed me and cleaned my room, but what I discovered is that men were also capable of great care, great tenderness, great motherliness, and it made gender disappear for me. As a Zen teacher, I wouldn't be able to have male students today if I felt otherwise. Because of the kindness of these men, I was able to see individuals for who they were, not what sex organs they have.

—*Darlene Cohen*

TRANSCENDENTAL REHAB

As a therapist and chaplain, I have worked with many populations, including people with AIDS, but presently I choose to work with felons, people who are definitely guilty, who have the criminal mind and intent. They are referred to me when the court and their therapists have given up, and I work with them to heal them of their criminality. Today I am working with people with whom I once said I couldn't work before—men who commit domestic violence, who attack women, who sexually abuse children. It's only recently that I've felt developed enough to work with such people. It's like facing down a demon energy, like dharma combat—very different work than helping a dying person or a grief-stricken family. At earlier times in my life I wasn't strong enough and I could be "had."

I remember one case of a man on parole who, while I was working with him, not only had a restraining order from his first wife but also stole money from his second wife, then beat her up. It threw our whole treatment into jeopardy because it meant that no good was coming of our relationship. So I had to negotiate with the court and his therapists and convince them all that I had the confidence I could be effective with him. Otherwise he was facing life imprisonment. I had to make quite a case, but finally he was given partial imprisonment and let out twice a week for treatment.

He was a very scary guy. He had a tricky mind, very psychopathic. He justified violence. He had no sense of consequence and constantly blamed others. Everything was minimized and trivialized; it was always "the system" doing him in. But when you have this closing window of opportunity to save someone from a lifetime of imprisonment, you have to amass all your forces and try to put someone on alert, in touch with their true nature. And you have to do it with the clock ticking.

Before each of his sessions, I had to work up a sense of my own presence because sometimes I worked alone in the office. I would go through all my fantasies. There would be nihilistic fantasies—that this wasn't going to work—and fear fantasies—that he would do me bodily harm. It became clear that I needed to go to the deepest part of myself so I could instinctually become like a tiger—beyond thought. To do so I would have to rely on deep faith in my Zen training and in myself. I had to face the fact that if I wasn't enlightened, how could I enlighten anybody else? It certainly brings your practice to the edge.

Throughout our work together, I constantly brought him back to the fact that he was ruining his life and the lives of others. He finally realized he was facing life incarceration, and we made a contract together. Our goal was to keep him out of jail and unite him with his children, but in order to do so I would have to move in on him—and hard. Furthermore, he had to agree not to fight the women's suits against him. Initially he went for it and then we started confronting his deviations, evasions, and rationalizations. I had to be surefooted like a mountain goat because he was trying to throw me off every second. I had to clearly see his mental habits but also believe that there was a being beyond all who was not caught up in that. I had to put all my faith in his deeper self; otherwise he would have nothing to drop into, just his bag of tricks.

We never talked about Buddhism, but I considered what we were doing a meditation. A turning point came for him that was also a simultaneous crisis for me. At the time, I was trying to work with my fear of what he had clearly laid out as his evil intent to hurt me. He was due to arrive for a session. He would come from the elevator and down a long hall with a dark corner at the end. I came out a few minutes early and stood there. When he rounded the corner, I didn't move as he came down this very long hall. The light was toward my office. Our eyes met and neither of us took our eyes off each other for the length of that walk. Worlds passed before my eyes, and in that moment, I corrected my own perception out of the fear realm. When he saw he had to meet me where I was, something happened in his eyes.

That was the beginning of a deep shift, and six months later he was judged by the court and various therapists as being on his way to cure. Finally he confessed to the court, didn't defend himself, took his punishment, and reconciled in a friendly way with his first wife, so much so that he was allowed Sunday dinner with his children and their mother once a week at his parents' house. So here was somebody who had been hell-bent on destroying himself and others and was instead plucked out of the fire. Perhaps more accurately, I stood in that fire with him. It was just at the edge of my skill level and tolerance, and through the whole work I could feel my own self burning.

—*Diane Martin*

INVINCIBLE FAITH

As long as I can remember I have had the desire to help others. I remember when I was about seven years old, I saw some older kids throwing stones at an animal. I don't know how, but I managed to frighten them away with a big wooden stick. When I discovered the animal was a snake, a long one, but not poisonous, I put it on the stick and brought it home. It had some wounds so I went to get some medicine to clean it up. Then I applied some green clay to help the wound heal quicker. When I realized the clay would fall off the moment the snake moved, I tried putting a bandage around its neck, whereupon it moved its head and bit me, then slowly moved away. (I still have the scar on my finger!) Even at seven, however, I never thought the snake was bad for biting me. I understood even then that it was only because I had caused it some pain.

Years later, when I was in South India, I was looking after a small dispensary. At noontime, some kids arrived, helping a very pale and bleeding teenager to walk into the main room. We put him on the examination table and discovered he had a very deep wound on his cheek. His friends told me he had fallen down on a broken window. I checked his blood pressure and it was very low. Other Tibetan people wanted to send him to a hospital, but I knew he didn't have more than ten or fifteen minutes to live. I'm not a surgeon, but on my own I've learned a few things about basic surgery, mainly from books. So it became clear for me that I had to try something.

First, I made a quick but very intense prayer. Within a few minutes, I gave him general anesthesia. My first goal was to stop the bleeding. On a hand or a foot, it's easy, you have plenty of time. But on the face, where do you put the tourniquet? As soon as I put a compress on the wound and took it away, it was full of blood. It took me a few seconds to understand that I had to follow the "flow of blood" to understand from where it could originate. People usually don't understand what I mean, but at that moment I could see clearly the "whirl" of red cells. Finally I found the artery and everything calmed down a bit. The biggest danger was over. It then took me two hours to stitch the muscles. (I asked someone to bring me my anatomy book because there are so many muscles there!) The boy woke up about one hour after I had completely closed everything. One hour later, his blood pressure returned to normal. I went home, exhausted, but happier than I have ever felt. Without a doubt, I knew also that my deep faith had saved that kid.

—*Ven. Lama Shenphen*

> The more we truly desire to benefit others, the greater the strength and confidence we develop and the greater the peace and happiness we experience.
>
> —*His Holiness the Dalai Lama*

GIFT OF FREEDOM

A juvenile delinquent who ended up in San Quentin State Prison at the age of nineteen for multiple robberies, Jarvis Jay Masters was later sentenced to death for conspiring to murder a prison guard. He is presently on Death Row awaiting appeal. During his incarceration, he encountered Buddhism and began a devout practice of meditation under the tutelage of the Tibetan master H. E. Chagdud Tulku. His memoirs, *Finding Freedom: Writings from Death Row,* from which this passage is excerpted, is an unforgettable story of both the horrors and boredom of prison life and the opportunity for spiritual salvation it affords.

I was walking out on the exercise yard last week, along the fence, staring up at the beautiful clear sky. It was a gorgeous day. Then something frightening happened: someone got stabbed on the adjacent yard. In the gunmen's tower, prison guards were racking rounds into their rifles. They were shooting at two guys' scuffling and fighting and trying to kill each other. I knew immediately that someone was going to die. Either the guards or one of these two prisoners would be responsible for taking a human being's life.

The tower gunmen ordered everyone facedown on the ground as they swung their fully loaded rifles around the three adjacent yards. I didn't know what to think. Since I didn't hear any gunshots, I figured the two guys must have stopped fighting. At least the gunmen had been saved from taking someone's life. But what about the prisoner who had been stabbed? Was he dead? What had I been thinking about before all this happened? Why am I lying here like this? Is this all real? Shit! How long can I go on trying to be a Buddhist in this prison culture that has me lying facedown? Who am I kidding?

Just as I thought my head would explode from so many flashing thoughts, I locked onto a single idea; how some people in this world have only a tragic five seconds to put their entire lives in order before they die—in a car crash or in some other sudden way. I realized that what really matters isn't where we are or what's going on around us, but what's in our hearts while it's happening.

I used to feel I could hide inside my practice, that I could simply sit and contemplate the raging anger of a place like this, seeking inner peace through prayers of compassion. But now I believe love and compassion are things to extend to others. It's a dangerous adventure to share with them in a place like S.Q. yet I see now that we become better people if we can touch a hardened soul, bring joy into someone's life, or just be an example for others, instead of hiding behind our silence.

The key is in using what we know. This calls for lots of practice. There is this vast space in life to do just that, both as a practitioner and as someone who walks around the same prison yard as everyone else in this place. I've learned how to accept responsibility for the harm I've caused others by never letting myself forget the things I did and by using those experiences to help others understand where they lead.

—*Jarvis Jay Masters*

> Loving-kindness is the wish that others will experience happiness and find the causes of this happiness. All beings long for happiness, but hardly any achieve it. So to wish them as much happiness as possible and to wish that they may find the causes of happiness is called "loving-kindness." Loving-kindness has immeasurable qualities. If you have this love deep within your being, you naturally benefit others. And there is no way that any kind of evil influence can harm you, for compassion is the most powerful weapon against negative forces.
>
> — *Dilgo Khyenste Rinpoche*

HUGGING MEDITATION

One normally doesn't associate physical affection with Buddhist meditation practice, which is why the following passage by the Vietnamese monk and meditation teacher Thich Nhat Hanh is so extraordinary.

Hugging meditation is a practice I invented. In 1966, a woman poet took me to the Atlanta Airport and then asked, "Is it all right to hug a Buddhist monk?" In my country we are not used to expressing ourselves that way, but I thought, "I am a Zen teacher. It should be no problem for me to do that." So I said, "Why not?" and she hugged me. But I was quite stiff. While on a plane, I decided that if I wanted to work with friends in the West, I would have to learn the culture of the West, so I invented hugging meditation.

Hugging meditation is a combination of East and West. According to the practice, you have to really hug the person you are hugging. You have to make him or her very real in your arms, not just for the sake of appearances, patting him on the back to pretend you are there, but breathing consciously and hugging with all your body, spirit and heart. Hugging meditation is a practice of mindfulness. "Breathing in, I know my dear one is in my arms, alive. Breathing out, she is so precious to me." If you breathe deeply like that, holding the person you love, the energy of care, love, and mindfulnesss will penetrate into that person and she will be nourished and bloom like a flower.

At a retreat for psychotherapists in Colorado, we practiced hugging meditation, and one retreatant, when he returned home to Philadelphia, hugged his wife at the airport in a way he had never hugged her before. Because of that, his wife attended our next retreat in Chicago. To be really there, you only need to breathe mindfully, and suddenly both of you become real. It may be one of the best moments in your life.

—*Thich Nhat Hanh, from* Teachings on Love

Indeed there is not a single sentient being in the universe who has not been our father or mother at some time or another.

— *Dilgo Khyentse Rinpoche*

TRANSFORMING HORROR

Early in the last decade, Thich Nhat Hanh organized a retreat for American veterans of the Vietnam War. Many of them—women and men—were struggling with anger, self-loathing, and guilt, and deeply desired to find a way out of their personal hell. In this passage from his book *Teachings on Love,* the Vietnamese monk draws upon deep wells of forgiveness to teach veterans a way to heal their painful memories.

Another veteran told us that almost everyone in his platoon had been killed by the guerillas. Those who survived were so angry that they baked cookies with explosives in them and left them alongside the road. When some Vietnamese children saw them, they ate the cookies, and the explosives went off. They were rolling around the ground in pain. Their parents tried to save their lives, but there was nothing they could do. That image of the children rolling on the ground, dying because of the explosives in the cookies, was so deeply ingrained on this veteran's heart, that now, twenty years later, he still could not sit in the same room with children. He was living in hell. After he had told this story, I gave him the practice of Beginning Anew.

Beginning Anew is not easy. We have to transform our hearts and our minds in very practical ways. We may feel ashamed, but shame is not enough to change our heart. I said to him, "You killed five or six children that day? Can you save the lives of five or six families today? Children everywhere in the world are dying because of war, malnutrition, and disease. You keep thinking about the five or six children that you killed in the past, but what about the children who are dying now? You still have your body, you still have your heart, you can do many things to help children who are dying in the present moment. Please give rise to your mind of love, and in the months and years that are left to you, do the work of helping children." He agreed to do it, and it has helped him transform his guilt.

—*Thich Nhat Hanh*

The only peace it is meaningful to speak about is world peace.

— *His Holiness the Dalai Lama*

ANTIDOTE TO PANIC

Recently I was scheduled to have the medical test known as a colonoscopy. It is an extremely invasive procedure into the most intimate parts of one's body and therefore frightening for most people. For that reason patients are usually asked to bring someone with them so they can be accompanied home. Unfortunately, due to the timing of my procedure, I didn't have anybody to come with me, so I was already feeling quite vulnerable from the start. On top of that, my veins are quite small and my doctor had a terrible time inserting the IV for the anesthesia. For some reason, my memory of the day is still fresh, as if it is happening now. Strapped to the gurney and dressed only in a patient's gown, I do everything not to squirm, but he misses . . . first time . . . second . . . third. The needle is huge and the pain is excruciating. As he taps up and down my arm looking for a vein, I can feel his nervousness through his finger. Seeing me break out in a sweat, he asks if I've brought somebody with me. Tears well up in my eyes. "That's okay," he says unconvincingly, "you'll be fine." Finally, on the fifth try, the needle connects with a vein. I'm about to exhale in relief when I hear him yell to his attendant, "Okay, hit the *music.*" At this point, the loudest, most raucous, most offensive rock music blasts through the room. I'm stunned. I can't believe I have to ask him to turn it off.

"I can't," he says, strapping on his mask. "This is the way I work."

I'm just outraged. Strapped down like a prisoner, I feel the heavy-metal beat rattle my bones and I feel like I've entered hell. Sweat pours down my face and I begin to shake uncontrollably. Never before have I felt so trapped in a nightmare, and worse, there is absolutely no escape. In less than a minute, I will probably be unconscious. I actually feel like I am about to be executed, poison draining into my system through the IV. I'm completely on the edge of panic and the only thing I have on my side is my own mind. And then, squeezed by this physical, mental, and emotional claustrophobia, something shifts, and maybe *because* I am in such an intense state of suffering, I suddenly open to an awareness where I feel not just my suffering but also the suffering of umpteen billion beings in the world who have gone through this same kind of experience. I think of my friend Sylvan who endured thousands of IVs during the long years of his diabetes. My father and mother, my brothers, before surgeries. Millions I have never met who face trauma, fear, helplessness, every day. The room feels full of spirits. Then somewhere in me, almost as if I had been rumbling in the dark for eons looking for it, a prayer arises in my mind, one taught to me so long ago by my masters: *May all those who have this same kind of suffering never have to experience it again. May this suffering I am enduring release them from their agony.*

And then I am out cold. My next memory is the nurse telling me it's over. The procedure has gone fine, and after the IV episode there is almost no pain. I get up, dress, and take the subway home by myself. The whole episode is almost like a dream. But the experience taught me something I will never ever forget—how easily distress can arrive, how helpless sentient beings are, and how entrenched prayer must be in our mindstreams so we can use it when we need it.

—*Pamela Bloom*

THE HEART THAT GOES ON

I was running a wellness community in California when I met an oncologist who happened to be the chemotherapist of the comedian Gilda Radner. Radner was struggling with ovarian cancer, and he thought my background as a psychotherapist and meditator could help her. From the moment we met, I was deeply moved by her sweetness and open-heartedness. During the course of working with me, she would often talk about her symptoms as if what she was experiencing was unique. One day I pointed out to her that I was working at a place where these things were rather common, shared by a lot of people. She wasn't alone. Gilda paused for a moment and then said, "So—I'm boring you?" We both laughed.

When Gilda finally decided to come to our center and tell her story, she found the experience hugely liberating. Slowly she came to learn how to live with the ambiguity of living and dying, and deeply grasped the teaching I shared with her from my first Buddhist master, Suzuki Roshi—that in the beginner's mind there are many possibilities, but in the expert's mind, only a few. Not being "expert" in knowing the moment of her death left her free to live her life. Often she and her husband, Gene Wilder, talked about establishing a similar center on the East Coast. She even tried to recreate a cancer support community in her own living room, but it couldn't be done. It lacked a structure and a facilitator. To work, it had to be something more than just people sitting around and talking about their emotions.

About a year after her death, a group of people, including her husband, Gene, the TV movie critic Joel Siegel, and the actor Mandy Patinkin, called and suggested I try to start something in New York. When they asked me how much money I would need, I naively guessed, "Oh, maybe ten thousand dollars." Armed with another ten thousand that I borrowed from a friend, I gave up my home and life in California, which I had enjoyed for twenty years, and took a tiny apartment sight-unseen in Manhattan. Really, all I had was a dinosaur Macintosh computer and the ideas that had been percolating in my mind and heart for many years as a psychotherapist working with families and cancer. But from the first moment, I encountered what many of us would later call "Gilda's magic," because I miraculously found fervently devoted sponsors and supporters, and the blessings of people who were already doing complementary things. Today, after much hard work, there are eight Gilda's Clubs in America and six more to open this year, with another fifteen to twenty in development. We now call it Gilda's Club Worldwide.

What I really love about Gilda's Club is that it was completely informed by my Buddhist training, and yet most people involved have no idea of that. Here's how it works. People meet at Gilda's Club as a community, a sangha. They gather together to support one another as they learn how to live with cancer, whatever the outcome. Our stated philosophy is that the real expert on living with cancer, socially and emotionally, is within themselves; it comes from their direct experience. And yet this is something they can share with others—what I call our "collective wisdom." And this sangha includes husbands, wives, children, family, friends, neighbors, clergy, your accountant, your dog, anybody in your world who is open to exploring what it means to be living with cancer. Every aspect of the program is designed to reinforce this philosophy. And there's no charge for anything.

I remember one woman who became a "member"of Gilda's Club very secretively, having spoken to virtually no one about the fact that she had cancer and was in treatment. This shame was a significant part of her world, but eventually she entered into many of our activities and made a lot of friends. The course of her disease went up and down, but what constantly grew was the sense of herself as person capable of living with cancer, and living well. Her favorite activity was the arts workshop. One day one of our national sponsors was looking for celebrities to create a special tie promotion and I said, "We have celebrities right here in our workshop, people who are living every day with cancer and are creating beautiful works of art." One of her drawings was chosen and ended up on a tie, and her glamorous photograph, looking happy and proud, was reproduced on the hangtag, a tag that went out to over eight hundred national retail stores, identifying her as a member of Gilda's Club living with cancer. Afterward she came to me and said, "I was in the closet when I came to Gilda's Club and now I'm shouting from the rooftop. I don't know what the outcome will be, but I know now that I can live with cancer every day—and lots of times *wonderfully.*"

Gilda's brother told me that this work is perhaps even more Gilda's legacy than her comedy because through her inspiration, thousands of people are now giving and receiving social and emotional support that they never would have had. Gilda used to say that having cancer was like being in an elite club she would rather not belong to. That's why we called it Gilda's Club: We start with a laugh and learn how to live, together.

—Joanna Bull

ORIGINS OF PEACE

All of my early life I decried violence in the world. My family was Jewish and in the late forties talk of the Holocaust and of missing relatives in Europe was occasional dinner table conversation. The recurrent question for me was, How could people act so inhumanely toward one another? As the years passed by, I became more and more committed to nonviolence. At the same time, as I judged world violence, I became increasingly distant and judgmental of my own darker side.

The year 1960 found me away from home for the first time and committed to doing work for peace. I had never considered that the origins of peace must lie within myself. When I first was involved in nonviolent direct action, I was just eighteen. In the training, we were asked to look at our own anger. I remember thinking, "No, I won't be angry! I'll be kind and loving." We were to begin picketing a facility that built nuclear submarines. I'd promised to be physically nonviolent, but I knew nothing of what nonviolence meant. My promise was easily made since I thought it was only about restraining myself against striking back, and I thought that would be simple.

I was picketing in a place where there'd been no previous violence. A man who was a little drunk and feeling belligerent approached me. He was angry; we were threatening his job. He pushed me, then slapped me, not hard enough to do any real damage, but enough to scare me. As he pushed I fell to the ground and protected my face as I'd been taught. He kicked at me, again hurting my pride far more than my body, mostly taunting me.

I lay there on the ground, not hitting back but hating him. I remember the feel of it—scratchy gray concrete sidewalk and sharp pebbles that poked into the soft palm flesh, the one icy puddle that soaked my knees, the dull thud of his boot against my shoulder. I felt so much fear and anger. It wasn't just anger at him but at my own response. I'd promised to be nonviolent, to be loving. I *was* loving! Where was all this anger coming from? Finally people pulled him off. His final words were "I'll see you next week if you're not too scared."

Scared? I was terrified, not of him but of the potential for violence I suddenly saw in myself. I explored that fear during the week, but the next Saturday the same scene repeated itself and the same fear and anger arose.

We played this out week after week—a little stage show. Soon we had an audience gathering on Saturday afternoons, coming to expect our little drama! Each week I lay there hating him, hating myself even more because I was supposed to be loving and nonviolent.

I began to see the roots of my anger, that I wasn't angry at him for pushing or kicking me but for reflecting my own helplessness and rage so clearly. Slowly I found some compassion for myself, lying there trembling on the ground. I began to allow my anger, to see that even with that anger I didn't have to retaliate. I started to respect myself for that.

I saw that my anger masked fear, not of being hurt, because he clearly wasn't going to really hurt me, but fear of losing control. Anger was a way of feeling safe, moving into the old dualities of right/wrong, good/bad. If I was "good" and he was "bad," then I didn't have to explore my own potential for violence. I could just safely blame another. But if I was also angry, where did safety lay? As I opened to these fears in myself and found acceptance of them, I also began to relate more openly to his fear. Suddenly, instead of an opponent, I saw a mirror of myself, a being suffering and filled with fear.

Then it stopped being his fear or mine and was just fear. As I found the ability to be present with my own anger without judgment, I could also be present with his, no longer his or mine, just anger. There we were, doing this dance together. I felt my heart open in compassion for us both.

The first time I understood this it was like walking from dark shadow to bright sunlight. I lay there on the ground, feeling his feet against my head and ribs, and suddenly I loved him. I'm not saying there was no longer anger, but it was more just the continuing reverberations of anger in the body, taking their time to fade away. Simultaneously, there was loving spaciousness. There was no more judgment, just two people feeling fear together. A world feeling fear together! As my heart opened with this insight most of the anger dissolved. There wasn't anything left to fear.

As that change occurred in me he felt it. For weeks this had been a wordless encounter. Suddenly he stopped. I lay there for a few moments and then looked up, making eye contact for the first time. He spoke, "Why do you keep coming back?" Our eyes held one another. He offered his hand and helped me to my feet.

The door of communication opened. My opening to my own anger had helped him start to accept his own emotions. We went off to a small restaurant to talk together, the two of us and several of our friends. With the barriers of judgment lowered, we began to actually hear each other. For the first time I heard his fears about losing his job, not being able to support his family. For the first time he truly heard and considered our views. Lessening our attachment to our own tunnel vision, communication grew, and in a constantly expanding group, we began to meet regularly to talk. Rather than remaining two opposing forces, we became a group of individuals, each with his or her own concerns, working together to resolve our fears and pain.

—*Barbara Brodsky*

As long as you do not change your mind, there will always be an enemy to harm you.

—*Lama Thubten Zopa Rinpoche*

For as long as space endures
And sentient beings suffer
May I also remain
To dispel the world's sorrows.

—*Shantideva*

Directing *the* Mind, Defrosting *the* Heart:

Meditations for Developing Compassion

METTA PRACTICE

The practice of Metta, or loving-kindness, is a specific meditation that can be used to cultivate not only a calm, concentrated mind but also the quality of loving-kindness itself. Simple and direct, the practice is appropriate for use by anyone regardless of their religious affiliation, for it is based purely on love. Its power lies not in the mindless repetition of phrases but in the deep connection one makes within the heart to the words' deeper meaning. In a sense, the practice of Metta as described below turns the mind to the possibility that the sentiments expressed will one day open the heart and truly become one's own. By repeating these words in a slow, graceful, purposeful way (and making up your own as the intention arises), over time the practice will take on a life of its own—*your* life—and begin to penetrate the deep resistances that keep us from acting at all times from our true compassionate loving selves.

It is ideal if you can do this practice in a quiet place for about fifteen to twenty minutes daily over a period of several months. At first this meditation may feel mechanical or awkward, or it may even bring up feelings of irritation or anger. If this happens, don't despair. The masters say that the arousal of negativity is a good sign, for it is as if the cleansing winds of loving-kindness are blowing up any dirt or dust that has accumulated over years and eons of forgetfulness. Metta can be seen as a form of house-cleaning, so when difficult emotions arise, it is important to be patient and kind toward yourself. Receive whatever arises in a spirit of friendliness and kind affection. In time, you may find this practice is actually becoming your dearest friend, supporting you through the most difficult situations in silent waves of love.

To begin the practice in a formal way, sit in a comfortable position. If you are sitting in a chair, feel your feet flat on the floor and sit in a stable position without leaning forward or back. Let your body relax and your breathing find its natural balance. Let go, as best you can, of any worries or preoccupations. You may keep your eyes open or closed, but if you practice with them open, focusing softly into space, you may discover over time that the practice translates more easily into daily life. When you feel ready, begin to recite silently to yourself the following phrases directed first toward yourself. You begin with yourself because the Buddha teaches that without loving oneself it is almost impossible to love others: *May I be well. May I be happy. May I be free from suffering. May I be filled with loving-kindness. May I be filled with joy. May I be at peace and at ease.*

As you say these phrases, focus on the area around your heart and allow the meaning and sense of the words to penetrate into your very being, blood, bones, and sinews. Allow to arise the confidence that through the repetition of these words, the more you allow yourself to be well, to be happy, so shall you be. As you recite these words inwardly, you may also wish to visualize yourself as a young child being embraced by your mother, or held sweetly in the arms of the Divine, however you picture its face. You may also begin to find your breathing slowing down and an inclination to synchronize the phrases with the exhalation. Allow whatever comes up naturally to soothe and calm you. Repeat the phrases again and again, letting the feeling waves of warmth, affection, and goodwill permeate your entire body and mind.

Practice this meditation repeatedly for a number of weeks until the sense of loving-kindness for yourself begins to come easily.

When it feels time, expand the meditation gradually to include loving-kindness toward others. After concentrating on your own happiness for a while, choose someone in your life whom you deeply love or care for, someone for whom "wishing well" is not a chore. Picture that person vividly before you in your mind's eye, sensing and feeling his or her presence. Then carefully recite the same phrases: *May you be well. May you be happy. May you be free from suffering. May you be filled with loving-kindness. May you filled with joy. May you be at peace and at ease.*

When loving-kindness for your closest loved one is developed, begin to include others in your life: friends, neighbors, community members, citizens of other countries, the animal kingdom, the whole earth and its beings. Then you can even experiment by including the most difficult people in your life, wishing that they too be filled with loving-kindness. Be sure to include those in the world who have no food, no shelter, the lonely and the forgotten, wishing all to be happy, well, and at peace. Even though you may not know specific names, choose a category of people—the homeless, people with AIDS, victims of war and social crisis, both the persecuted and the persecutors—and concentrate sending them Metta for a period of time. With some practice a steady sense of loving-kindness can develop in you, and in the course of fifteen or twenty minutes you will be able to include many beings in your meditation, moving from yourself to a benefactor and loved ones, to all beings everywhere. End your meditation session by changing the phrase to: *May all be well. May all be happy. May all be free from suffering. May all be filled with loving-kindness. May all be filled with joy. May all be at peace and at ease.*

Then you can graduate to practicing Metta everywhere. You can use this meditation waiting in traffic, on the subway, in doctor's offices, in a thousand other circumstances. As you silently practice this loving-kindness it will slowly become a positive habit of mind, replacing other habits of negativity. If you practice this meditation silently in the very midst of people, you will find yourself feeling an immediate connection with others. The power of loving-kindness will calm your life and help you stay centered in your heart.

TONGLEN: GIVING AND RECEIVING

The Tibetan practice of Tonglen is one of the most powerful and useful practices of compassion in all of Buddhism. As Sogyal Rinpoche writes in *The Tibetan Book of Living and Dying,* "When you feel yourself locked in yourself, Tonglen opens you to the truth of the suffering of others; when your heart is blocked, it destroys those forces that are obstructing it; and when you feel estranged from the person who is in pain before you, or bitter or despairing, it helps you to find within yourself and then to reveal the loving, expansive radiance of your own true nature."

In the essential Tonglen practice, we basically take on, through compassion, all the varied and sundry sufferings of beings—emotional, physical, and spiritual—and then offer them all our love, happiness, well-being, goodness, and peace of mind. And we do this through the medium of the breath: We breathe in their pain, their sorrow, their anger and their frustration, and we breathe out healing, fulfillment, and light. We begin with our own selves, breathing in our own pain and breathing out release. Then we gradually expand first to those toward whom we feel loving, then to those toward whom we feel neutral, and eventually to those toward whom we feel aversion. As you do the practice, equally applied to all three categories, you may discover that your own extreme emotions are beginning slowly to relax and that you actually become able to regard all beings with a sense of equanimity and impartiality.

What makes it possible for us as ordinary beings to make such a Bodhisattva gesture as take on the suffering of others is the innate presence of the "living Buddha" within. It is important to understand that we take on the suffering of others not as a martyr or to make ourselves sicker, but because we can actually afford to. In fact, it is very important to begin the practice of Tonglen by first flashing on that sense of the Divine, the living Buddha, Christ, our basic goodness *within,* so that we can then extend it to others. Otherwise the practice will deplete us and not be of value to others.

And yet, no matter how grand, how spacious our connection to that inner divinity is, we still feel ourselves vulnerable, tight, and resistant at times. Tonglen works with this very resistant, frozen self and uses it as the repository, the vehicle of contact to receive other people's suffering. Tonglen asks us to exchange ourselves, our suffering, for the suffering of others. And in the act of exchanging, we discover that not only is our suffering lessened but the suffering of others also begins to be dispelled.

Tonglen is a formal practice and should be done ideally on a daily basis in a quiet place for at least twenty to thirty minutes. It is a wonderful meditation to do in the midst of life: on the subway, walking down the street, in the middle of the workday, wherever you come upon people and situations that call for a compassionate response. It is particularly helpful at the time of death, to be done both by the person dying and by those in loving attendance, whether in the room physically or in spirit.

There are many variations of Tonglen. Pema Chödrön offers several excellent tapes that provide explicit instructions and guided meditations that take you through the process. The following "interfaith" version is based partially on both the teachings of Sogyal Rinpoche as they appear in the book mentioned above and those of my first teacher, Chögyam Trungpa Rinpoche.

Before you begin this practice, sit quietly and bring your mind to a focused, gentle awareness in the present moment. If you practice any other form of meditation that stills the mind, now would be a good time to do it. As your thoughts settle, call to mind an image, situation, or object of devotion that stimulates your heart of compassion, that truly opens you and helps you to feel the warmth, the heat, the power of spacious love. (You might do Metta practice first.) Perhaps it is the feeling of being in your mother's arms as a child, or the loving care of a mentor or friend, perhaps the Sacred Heart of Jesus, or the blessed arms of the Divine Mother, even the face of a beloved pet who has touched you deeply. Then let that feeling of love, warmth, and compassion fill and flood every part of your own being until you feel strengthened, refreshed, and revitalized. For a moment, flash on the sense of your own being as open and pure and spacious as a perfectly blue sky.

Then imagine in front of you, as vividly and poignantly as possible, someone you care for who is suffering. Let the image of his or her suffering take full root in your mind's eye in all its vivid detail. See, hear, and smell her suffering, her pain, her private sorrows. Then as you feel your heart opening in compassion toward this person, visualize that all of his or her suffering on every level—physical, mental, and emotional—coalesces and manifests in the form of a hot, black, gritty smoke.

Then as you breathe in, imagine that this mass of black smoke dissolves with your in-breath into the very core of your own attachment to your limited self, to your very resistance to doing the practice, to the parts of your heart that are still frozen. See this black, gritty smoke destroy and dissolve the very last vestiges of your own happiness that you have been holding onto at the expense of others.

Now that your frozen heart has dissolved, imagine that your awakened heart, your inherent basic goodness, your bodhichitta, is gloriously uncovered and fully revealed. As you breathe out, imagine that you are sending out on the exhaling breath a brilliant, cooling light of joy, peace, happiness, and well-being to your friend in pain, and that this light destroys all his or her negative thoughts and entanglements, thus purifying the karma.

You can even imagine that your entire body and being has been transformed into a brilliant, radiant wish-fulfilling jewel—one that grants the deepest desires and wishes of all and provides exactly what he or she needs to heal. You can even imagine he or she is receiving all the bright and beautiful things in your life as you breathe out and let go of your attachment to them, for in truth you have an unlimited store of them.

As you do this practice, remember to keep your breathing calm and steady. If you find yourself overwhelmed or lost in negativity, go back to the first image of love and care you generated until you feel stable again. In fact, doing Tonglen using yourself as the object is an excellent way to begin this practice; then move on to someone suffering who is close to you, then those who have caused you suffering, and then eventually to all those in the world who suffer. As a number of stories in this book have described, the greatest power of Tonglen is felt when it is done in the most negative of situations, that is to say, Tonglen done for those against whom you hold the most intense hatred or aversion. With time, practice, and devotion, the teachings of the living Buddha assure us that we all can get to the level of Palden Gyatso, the Tibetan monk mentioned earlier in this book, who was able to withstand the electric shock of his torturers by totally engaging his mind in the compassion-building practice of Tonglen.

GLOSSARY

Bardo: The intermediate state between the end of one life and the rebirth of another. Bardo also refers to the intermediate period between birth and death, and between sleeping and waking. It also refers to the gap between thoughts.

Bodhi: Derived from the Sanskrit root *budh,* which means "to wake up" and "to blossom," and which also gives us the word "buddha." According to Khunu Rinpoche, an enlightened being is buddha ("awakened") because he or she has cut the continuum of ignorance, like a being who has awakened from sleep. And an enlightened being is "buddha" ("opened") because perfect knowledge has destroyed the state of being tightly squeezed shut and has opened awareness to what is to be known, like the petals of a fully blossomed lotus.

Bodhichitta: The Mind of Enlightenment. On the relative level, bodhichitta is the wish to attain Buddhahood for the sake of all beings, as well as the practice necessary to accomplish such. On the absolute level, it is the direct insight into the ultimate nature of self and phenomena—the union of emptiness and compassion, which is beyond conceptualization.

Bodhisattva: One who possesses bodhichitta; a future Buddha. The Bodhisattva is committed to the practice of compassion and the six transcendent perfections, has vowed to attain enlightenment for the sake of all beings, and delays personal enlightenment to save other beings first. The Tibetan translation of the term literally means "hero of the enlightened mind."

Dharma: The body of teaching, expounded by the Buddha Shakyamuni and other enlightened beings, that shows the way to enlightenment.

Geshe: A Tibetan term that literally means "spiritual friend." Currently the title is generally conferred in the Gelugpa tradition of Tibetan Buddhism on those who have successfully completed many years of monastic education and have attained a high degree of doctrinal learning.

Incarnated lama: Also known as a "tulku," this is a master who, having achieved a high level of enlightenment and fortified by a desire to save sentient beings, reincarnates in subsequent lives in order to continue his or her spiritual work. Though they usually never admit it, tulkus are often endowed with strong spiritual traits, such as brilliant minds, clairvoyance, and healing powers.

Karma: The law of cause and effect; the process whereby virtuous actions of body, speech, and mind lead to happiness and nonvirtuous ones lead to suffering. The actions of each sentient being are the causes that create the conditions of rebirth and the circumstances in that lifetime.

Karmapa: A lineage of incarnate Bodhisattvas or tulkus in the Tibetan Buddhist Kagyu tradition. Karmapas are thought to be the incarnation of the Bodhisattva Avalokiteshvara.

Mala: A string of beads (usually 108) used as a counting aid in mantra recitation in Tibetan and other traditions of Buddhism.

Mantra: Sacred words of power or incantation, the chanting of which is often used as a meditation device.

Metta (Sanskrit: *maitri*): According to His Holiness the Dalai Lama, if compassion is the will to share in the suffering of others, Metta, or loving-kindness, is the genuine aspiration that wishes others to be happy.

Merit: Good karma; the energy generated by positive actions of body, speech, and mind.

Nagarjuna: Considered one of the greatest human teachers of ancient India, he lived a mythical six hundred years from ca. 50 B.C.E. to 550 C.E. He was the trailblazer who established the Madhyamika system of philosophical tenets that influenced all lineages of Tibetan Buddhism. Among many other works, he authored *Precious Garland of Advice of a King* and a profound manual called *Wisdom.* He is also the founder of a major Tantric practice of the Esoteric Communion.

Rinpoche: Literally "most precious one," a form of address used in Tibetan Buddhism for incarnate lamas, abbots, and respected teachers.

Shakyamuni (563–483 B.C.E.): Fourth of the one thousand founding Buddhas of the present world age. Born a prince in the Shakya clan in north India, he was the founder of what came to be known as Buddhism, teaching both the sutra and tantra paths to liberation. The name Shakyamuni means "Sage of the Shakya Clan."

Shantideva: A great Indian master and member of the monastic university of Nalanda in the eighth century. His main work, the *Bodhicharyavatara* (Entrance to the Way of the Bodhisattva), is a masterpiece of eloquence, poetry, and insight about how to live life as a Bodhisattva.

Six perfections or *paramitas*: The six qualities perfected by a Bodhisattva on the path to buddhahood: generosity, ethical discipline, patience, diligence, meditative concentration, and wisdom. They are considered the guidelines for enlightened living within the Tibetan tradition.

Thangka: An elaborate sacred painting of various Buddhas and deities representing energies of one's own being that acts as a visual aid and inspiration for different meditation practices. Many Tibetan shrines have a thangka hanging on the wall behind them.

Tulku: Literally means "emanation body." A tulku is a reincarnate lama in the Tibetan tradition, one who has been formally recognized as the reincarnation of his or her predecessor. In this era, "tulkus" have been known to be reborn in the West.

Vipassana: Penetrative insight meditation that reveals the absence of inherent existence in both the mind and phenomena. Within the Theravadin tradition, it is specifically a form of meditation that focuses on the acute awareness of bodily and mental sensations.

ACKNOWLEDGMENTS

A book like this cannot come to fruition without the love, support, and inspiration of numerous people over many years. My full-hearted gratitude goes first to the late Chögyam Trungpa Rinpoche and his once-dharma heir Ösel Tendzin, who provided me with my first contact with the Buddhist teachings twenty-two years ago. I am particularly grateful for the concepts of spiritual warriorship and enlightened culture that Trungpa Rinpoche brought to the fore of Western consciousness and for his refined artistic sense, particularly in flower arranging and calligraphy. A special place in my heart is reserved for the late Ösel Tendzin, whose life in all its extremes remains a poignant reminder to us to wake up completely to our fullest potential.

My deepest gratitude also goes to Sogyal Rinpoche—for without the warmth, vibrancy, love, humor, and compassion of his teachings, this book would never have been written. As an interfaith minister and spiritual counselor, I have found the heart teachings in his book *The Tibetan Book of Living and Dying* to be extraordinarily helpful in working with people of all faiths as they face both the joyous and catastrophic events of their lives. For his generous offer to create a special calligraphy for this book, I am deeply and forever grateful. May the merit of this work bring him the strength, joy, and long life to continue his life's work benefiting beings.

The purest heart offering goes to the Indian master Mata Amritanandamyi (Ammachi), whose image of ceaselessly blessing thousands of people a day, taking each and everyone into her arms, will be etched forever in my heart as the archetype of compassion. Deep love and gratitude also goes to Mother Meera, Sri Aurobindo, and the Mother for invisible inspiration and guidance. Special thanks on the most innermost level goes to the late Dilgo Khyentse Rinpoche who has remained, most especially through the writing of this book, the deepest and most-abiding presence. I only need to glance at his visage, so beautifully portrayed by the Ven. Mathieu Ricard in his photo book *Journey through Enlightenment,* to see the very face of compassion itself.

I am also deeply grateful for the many masters who shared their hearts with me for this book. I will cherish the moments I spent with His Holiness Padma Norbu (Penor) Rinpoche as he remembered moments of compassion from his childhood, with deep thanks offered to Khenpo Tsewang Gyatso for translating and for sharing later his own story. Dr. Lene Handberg of Copenhagen, Denmark, was indefatigable in inspiring Tarab Tulku XI to open up and share stories, which she herself transcribed. Similar intervention was done by Ven. Thubten Lodrö, who introduced me to Lama Shenphen. The Ven. Segyu Choepel Rinpoche not only stopped to contribute a story in the midst of a very busy traveling schedule but also gave me a listening ear and a healing heart when I most needed it.

Both exiles from their respective countries for refusing to condone the abuse of human rights, the Ven. Thich Nhat Hanh and His Holiness the Dalai Lama stand as pillars of peace and compassion in a world gone awry. My deepest appreciation goes to both of them, not only for the unsurpassable model of their lives, but also for their kindness to allow me to use their words in this book. I offer my deepest prayers for their long lives—may they both be filled with health, strength, and joy to continue the profound missions they have set for themselves.

Gratitude goes again to Dr. Robert Thurman, for translating my interview with the Ven. Lungri Namgyal, former Abbot of the Gyüto Monastery, for an article on Tibetan chant that first appeared in *Parabola* magazine. Deep appreciation is also extended to Lama Surya Das for an hour of enchanting storytelling. An extra special acknowledgement to Barbara Brodsky for submitting writing samples that added so much to the depth to this book.

To all the contributors of this book, too numerous to mention here, I have nothing more valuable to offer than the sincerest prayer that your efforts to discover the roots of compassion in yourself will ultimately ignite an irresistible force that goes around the world. May you and those you love live to see it happen in your lifetime.

Many warm thanks to the Rigpa sangha, in particular Joanna Bull, Michael Damian, Mary Pratt, Kathy Rousseau, and Michel Rousseau, for very special moments of sharing and support. Special thanks also goes to Patrick Gaffney, Sogyal Rinpoche's senior-most student, and his assistant, Susie Godfrey. Unlimited appreciation is also extended to the sanghas of Vajradhatu and the Shambhala Center as well as the staff and students of the New Seminary in New York.

Loving thanks to Seppo Ed Farrey, for the inspiration of his life of service and for giving me the wonderful opportunity to work as a counselor at the Manhattan Center for Living founded by Marianne Williamson.

Special mention must also be made of Azusa Ammar, my Sangetsu flower arranging teacher, Rev. Larry Ammar, Rev.

Marco Rezende, and the Izunome Association and Johrei Fellowship. The teachings of the Japanese master Mokichi Okada have been instrumental in my life in realizing ways to benefit others, and I will forever be grateful. The opportunity to make a spiritual pilgrimage to Japan in the midst of writing this book is due to all of them.

From start to finish, the book would not have been realized without the shared vision of the staff at Conari Press, especially that trio of *dakinis*—Mary Jane Ryan, Brenda Knight, and Heather McArthur—who seem to have so much fun doing what they do. Their enthusiasm is infectious!

And to invisible helpers: Rev. Robina Courtin, Marcia Rose, Ven. Jinmyo Fleming, Kelsang Shraddha, Bill Hudson, Meri-Robin Monroe, Ven. Damcho Sangmo, Ani Ariana Krietemeyer, Wib Middleton, Kimberly Poppe, Andrea Shaw, and the Birkin Forest Monastery for behind-the-scene efforts. Special love to Sharon Azar-Hahn for the beautiful drawings of compassion goddesses that intermittently appeared on my office desk.

A heart full of appreciation goes to Joan Halifax, for agreeing to write the foreword of this book. Few women on the American scene of spiritual growth and personal development match her courage, brilliance, tenacity, and compassion to help others in their deepest times of distress. May her life and work for the benefit of others always be blessed!

Special love goes to the dearest of friends, some of whom read the manuscript at different stages and offered boats, barges, and million-dollar lifelines to cross the river of doubt and hesitation: Leon Fabrizzi, Marsha Woolf, Carla Flack, Dr. LiLi Wu, B. Bloom, Massimo Ferrari, Professor Takaya Kawabe, and especially to Faye Hamel Levey, for her empathy and eagle editorial eye.

Lastly, my deepest love and appreciation goes to the members of my family, each of whom in his or her own way realize compassion on a daily basis. My late father, Dr. Manuel G. Bloom, Sr., was one of the first dermatologists to offer treatment at leper colonies in the Deep South, and my brothers, Dr. Kim Bloom, M.D., and Dr. Kerry Bloom, D.D.S., continue to this day in the family tradition of unstintingly helping others. My mother, Mitzie Muntz Bloom, in her inimitable fashion, long ago mastered the art of thinking of others first. May all their dreams be realized and may the merit of this book return again and again to bless them and their families.

And finally, to the staff at *Guideposts*, thank you for showing me the power of the story.

Pamela Bloom

CONTRIBUTORS

Sharon Azar-Hahn, p. 46, has been a practitioner of meditation for over twelve years. A lover of all animals, she has dedicated her life to the rescue of dogs (and sometimes cats) in the New York City area. She is founder of W.O.O.F. (Wagging On and On Foundation) dedicated to stray dogs. For more information, call (212) 608-5909.

Barbara Brodsky, pp. 97, 146, has been practicing meditation since 1960 and teaching worldwide since 1989. Profoundly deaf for twenty-four years, she is the guiding teacher of Deep Spring Center in Ann Arbor, Michigan.

Joanna Bull, p. 141, has been a student of Buddhism since she first went to Tassajara Zen Mountain Center in 1969 to study with Suzuki Roshi. She sat zazen alone for ten years, looking for another master, until she discovered Sogyal Rinpoche and made an easy transition to the study of Tibetan Buddhism. A psychotherapist and trainer, she is the founder of Gilda's Club Worldwide.

Pema Chödrön, p. 66, is an American Buddhist nun and one of the foremost students of Chögyam Trungpa Rinpoche, the late renowned meditation master. She is director of Gampo Abbey, Cape Breton, Nova Scotia, the first Tibetan monastery in North America established for Westerners. A highly sought-after speaker, she is the author of *The Wisdom of No Escape, Start Where You Are,* and *When Things Fall Apart.*

Ven. Segyu Choepel Rinpoche, p. 24, was born in Brazil and recognized as a healer at the age of four. For twenty-one years he underwent various rigorous trainings and initiations, which qualified him as a master of spiritual healing. Seeking his true roots in Tibetan Buddhism, he moved to the United States in 1983 to study with Tibetan masters. Two years later, Ven. Jampal Shenpen, the 98th Ganden Tri Rinpoche (lineage holder of the Gelugpa tradition founded by Lama Tsongkhapa), identified him as the reincarnation of Dorje Zangpo, a sixteenth-century Tantric master, and in 1997 he was formally enthroned in the Segyu Lineage by the senior masters of Sed-Gyued Datsang Tantric Monastery. An ordained monk who trains under Ven. Khensur Lati Rinpoche, he is the founding director and head lama of the Healing Buddha Foundation in Sebastopol, California, and teaches around the world.

Darlene Cohen, p. 122, began sitting in 1970 and was ordained as a priest in the lineage of Suzuki Roshi in 1974. Richard Baker Roshi was her main teacher. Now a teacher at the San Francisco Zen Center, she is the author of *Arthritis: Stop Suffering, Start Moving* and *Finding a Joyful Life in the Heart of Pain.*

His Holiness the 14th Dalai Lama, Tenzin Gyatso, p. 71, is the head of state and spiritual leader of the Tibetan people. He lives today in Dharmasala, India, as the leader of the Tibetan government-in-exile. For his unstinting efforts in the fields of global peace and human rights, he has been honored worldwide by universities and institutions; in 1989 he received the Nobel Peace Prize. Among his numerous books are *The Good Heart, Ethics for the New Millennium,* and *The Art of Happiness.*

Michael Damian, p. 72, is a specialist in conflict management, currently working for a leading nonprofit foundation in New York City. He became a student of Sufi master Adnan Sarhan in 1979 and has been a student of Sogyal Rinpoche since 1987.

Lama Surya Das, pp. 85, 89, is an American poet, writer, and Tibetan Buddhist lama and meditation teacher who has spent over eight years in seclusion and over twenty-five years practicing with the great teachers of the major Tibetan Buddhist schools. He is the author of *The Snow Lion's Turquoise Mane: Wisdom Tales from Tibet, Awakening the Buddha Within,* and *Awakening to the Sacred: Creating a Spiritual Life from Scratch.* He is the founder and spiritual director of Dzogchen Foundation, which has its headquarters in Massachusetts. His Web site is www.dzogchen.org.

Armen Donelian, p. 115, is renowned as a solo pianist and bandleader in Europe, the Middle East, Japan, and North America and recently received a New Jersey State Council on the Arts 2000 Fellowship in Music Composition. He has played with Sonny Rollins, Chet Baker, Lionel Hampton, Billy Harper, Paquito D'Rivera, and others. He is the director of the Jazz in Armenia Project, an educational and artistic initiative hosted by the Yerevan State. His Web site is www.armenjazz.com.

Seppo Ed Farrey, p. 76, has been the Tenzo (head chef) at Dai Bosatsu Zendo in Livingston Manor, New York, since 1994. He was ordained a Rinzai Zen Buddhist monk on May 31, 1997, and has received many awards for his volunteer work. He is the author of *Three Bowls: Vegetarian Recipes from an American Zen Buddhist Monastery.*

Bernard Tetsugen Glassman Roshi, p. 28, is the founder and abbot of the Zen Community of New York, the Zen Center of Los Angeles, and the Zen Mountain Center in Idyllwild, California. He is also the cofounder of Zen Peacemaker Order, an international order of social activists. He began studying Zen in 1958, received ordination from Maezumi Taizan Roshi in 1970, and eventually received dharma transmission to become his spiritual successor in the White Plum sangha. His latest book is *Bearing Witness: A Zen Master's Lessons in Making Peace.*

Ven. Palden Gyatso, p. 55, was born in southern Tibet in 1933. He joined the Drepelung Loseling monastery and became an ordained monk at the age of nineteen, just as Tibet was being torn by political upheaval. Since his release from a Chinese prison in 1992, he has continued to struggle for the freedom of the hundreds of political prisoners still behind bars in Tibet. He is the author of *The Autobiography of a Tibetan Monk.*

Khenpo Tsewang Gyatso, p. 38, is an eminent Tibetan Buddhist scholar and His Holiness Penor Rinpoche's representative in the

United States. He is one the three senior-most khenpos (teaching scholars) at Namdrölling Monastery in Mysore, India.

Joan Halifax Roshi, Ph.D., p. ix, is a Buddhist teacher and anthropologist who has worked with individuals suffering from life-threatening illnesses since 1970. In 1990, she founded Upaya, a Buddhist study center in Sante Fe, New Mexico, dedicated to practices that foster right livelihood and whose programs include the Project on Being With Dying. She has practiced Buddhism since the late sixties and was ordained in 1976. In 1990, she received the Lamp transmission from Thich Nhat Hanh, and in 1997, she was ordained as a Soto and Peacemaker Priest by Tetsugen Roshi. Her books include *A Buddhist Life in America, Simplicity in the Complex, The Human Encounter with Death* (with Stanislav Grof), *The Fruitful Darkness, Shamanic Voices,* and *Shaman: The Wounded Healer.*

Ven. Thich Nhat Hanh, pp. 27, 135, 137, Zen master, peacemaker, and author of thirty-five books including *Living Buddha, Living Christ* and *Being Peace,* was nominated by Martin Luther King, Jr., for the Nobel Peace Prize. He lives in Plum Village, a meditation community in France that he founded, and travels worldwide teaching "the art of mindfulness."

Jeffrey Hopkins, Ph.D., p. 81, is Professor of Tibetan Studies at the University of Virginia and served as Director of the Center for South Asian Studies there. A leading scholar in Tibetan Buddhism, he has published countless articles and twenty-three books, including *The Tantric Distinction: A Buddhist's Reflections on Compassion and Emptiness.*

John F. Kennedy, Jr., p. 42, was the son of the thirty-fifth President of the United States and Jacqueline Kennedy Onassis. A former assistant district attorney of the State of New York, he was the founder of *George* magazine, which continues to provide political and social commentary on national and world events.

Sister Chân Không (True Emptiness), p. 53, was born in Vietnam in 1938. In 1964, she joined Zen Master Thich Nhat Hanh in founding the School for Youth for Social Service, which grew to an organization of over 10,000 young people organizing medical, educational, and agricultural facilities in rural Vietnam and rebuilding villages destroyed by the war. She lives in exile in Plum Village, Thich Nhat Hanh's community in southwestern France, where she is a dharma teacher, community leader, and social worker. She is author of *Learning True Love: How I Learned and Practiced Social Change in Vietnam.*

Master Jae Woong Kim, p. 92, is the foremost disciple of the late Master Sung Wook Back, the most prominent Korean Buddhist teacher of the twentieth century. He is the head of the Diamond Monastery in Korea and travels frequently to the U.S. to give teachings. He is the author of *Polishing the Diamond, Enlightening the Mind: Reflections of a Korean Buddhist Master.*

P'nina Macher, p. 112, was born in Atlanta, Georgia, and received a master's degree in human resources from Georgia State University. She has worked as a consultant in hospitals and as a city planner, occupational therapist, Feldenkreis praciti-tioner, and psychotherapist. She first met the dharma through Chögyam Trungpa Rinpoche in 1978 and has been a student of Penor Rinpoche for five years.

Diane Martin, p. 125, is a Soto Zen priest and Ph.D. clinical psychologist specializing in felon offenders. She was ordained by Yvonne Rand with whom she has studied Tibetan Buddhism. She is the founder of the Udumbara Sangha, which, besides meditation, offers a chaplaincy track for work in hospitals and prisons. For more information, contact Udumbara Sangha, 501 Sherman Avenue, Evanston, IL 60202; (947)475-3264.

Jarvis Jay Masters, p. 131, is a convicted felon on Death Row in San Quentin State Prison. Through a campaign supported by sangha members, his case is presently on appeal. He is the author of the critically acclaimed memoir *Finding Freedom: Writings from Death Row.*

Ven. Lungri Namgyal, p. 118, is the former Abbot of the Gyuto monastery in Bodhila, India, one of the fountainheads of the Gelugpa lineage of Tibetan Buddhism and known worldwide for its strong Tantric chant tradition. Presently he is the director of centers throughout Europe.

Kate O'Neill, M.Ed., p. 41, has been practicing Vipassana and Zen meditation since 1986 and was ordained into Thich Nhat Hanh's Order of Interbeing in 1992. She lives in northern New Mexico where she is a counselor, teacher, painter, and writer.

Patrul Rinpoche (1808–87), p. 22, was one of the greatest Tibetan teachers of the nineteenth century. Famous for his precise and direct style, he shunned high monastic position and pursued instead the life of a homeless wanderer, writing his classic text, *The Words of My Perfect Teacher,* in a rustic hermitage under an overhanging rock.

Padma Norbu (Penor) Rinpoche, p. 88, is founder and Chief Rinpoche of Palyul Namdrölling Monastery in Mysore, South India, home to 1,800 monks with branches throughout the world. He is the eleventh throneholder of the Palyul mother monastery and is now serving as Supreme Head of the Nyingma School of Tibetan Buddhism. He is considered to be an emanation of the great Indian Pandit Vimalamitra who brought the Vajrayana teachings to Tibet with Guru Padmasambhava.

Michel Rousseau, pp. 64, 69, met the Buddhist teachings over twenty years ago. He has been a student of Dilgo Khyentse Rinpoche, Nyoshul Khenpo Rinpoche, and Sogyal Rinpoche. He is married and lives in Long Island.

Julia Russell, p. 56, was born in New Jersey in 1951. A completely self-taught artist, she discovered a natural ability for visually expressing the various spiritual traditions she encountered on her travels around the world. Specializing now in iconic art, her work has been shown in New York City and most recently at the Cathedral of St. John the Divine. She has practiced meditation for over twenty-five years.

Sharon Salzberg, p. 63, has been practicing Buddhist meditation for over twenty-five years. She is a cofounder of the Insight Meditation Society and has taught meditation at Buddhist centers around the world. She is the author of *A Heart as Wide as the World: Living with Mindfulness, Wisdom, and Compassion, Lovingkindness: The Revolutionary Art of Happiness,* and *Voices of Insight.*

Ven. Lama Shenphen, p. 129, was born in France in 1969. In 1985 he entered Nalanda, a Tibetan monastery in France, and he received full ordination as a monk by His Holiness the Dalai Lama at the age of twenty one. For his efforts in establishing four humanitarian missions to Tibetan refugee camps in southern India, he was awarded the "Servir" prize by a Rotary Club of France. Presently director of Zung-Jug-Ling Center on the island of Paros in Greece, he receives visitors for retreat, teachings, and healing. See www.users.otenet.gr/~dzl.

Sogyal Rinpoche, p. 23, is the author of *The Tibetan Book of Living and Dying,* which has sold more than a million copies around the world. Born in Tibet in 1948, he was raised by Jamyang Khyentse Chökyi Lodrö, one of the greatest masters of this century, who recognized him as the reincarnation of Terton Sogyal, a Dzogchen master and discoverer of hidden texts. He eventually studied comparative religion at Cambridge University in England and served as translator to His Holiness Dudjom Rinpoche in the West. He has founded numerous centers in Europe and North America, under the name Rigpa Fellowship, and is much in demand as a speaker around the world, particularly on topics having to do with death and dying. See www.rigpa.org.

Sylvia Somerville, p. 100, has been a student of Jetsunma Akhön Norbu Lhamo for over twenty years. She presently lives in Sedona, Arizona.

Tarthang Tulku, p. 30, was born in eastern Tibet, the son of an incarnate lama and village doctor. He received intensive Buddhist training from some of the greatest masters of his age and has devoted his life to integrating psychology, science, and the humanities with Buddhist thought. From 1962 to 1968, he taught philosophy at Sanskrit University in India. For the last thirty years, he has taught in the United States. He is the author of more than fifteen books and the founder of Dharma

Publishing and Dharma Press, Nyingma Institutes, Odiyan Country Center, and the World Peace Ceremony.

Ven Thubten Lodrö, p. 82, was born in France and became an ordained monk in the Gelugpa lineage of Tibetan Buddhism in the early nineties. He has worked with Lama Shenphen on the island of Paros in Greece in the establishment of a retreat center there.

Orgyen Tobgyal Rinpoche, p. 59, was born to an ancient family lineage of Buddhist gurus and yogis and is recognized as an incarnate lama from the Chokling Tersar tradition of the Nyingma School. Known for his encyclopedic knowledge of Buddhist history and practices as well as his mastery of Vajrayana rituals, he is considered by many young lamas as the bridge between conservative and liberal traditions. He played the role of the "geko" in the film *The Cup*.

Karma Lekshe Tsomo, p. 102, received ordination as a Buddhist nun with His Holiness the Gyalwang Karmapa in 1977 and full ordination in Korea in 1982. An instructor at Chaminade University and an affiliate at East-West Center in

Honolulu, she holds M.A. degrees in Asian studies and Asian religion from University of Hawai'i at Manoa, and is a doctoral candidate in Comparative Philosophy. She is secretary of Sakyadhita: International Association of Buddhist Women and director of Jamyang Choling, a network of eight Buddhist education programs for women in the Indian Himalayas. A highly regarded videographer and widely published writer, she has most recently written *Innovative Women in Buddhism: Swimming Against the Stream*.

Tarab Tulku Rinpoche, p. 106, is a Tibetan lama and the eleventh incarnation of Tarab Tulku. Educated in Tibet at the University of Drepung Monastery, he received the Geshe Lharampa degree in Buddhist philosophy and psychology. In the sixties, he was invited to join Copenhagen University and the Royal Library by Prince Peter of Denmark, where he has remained as research librarian and lecturer. Extensively published in scholarly journals, he has established Tarab Institutes in Paris, Vienna, Budapest, Munich, Brussels, Helsinki, Stockholm, and Copenhagen.

Lama Choedak Yuthok, p. 109, is the founder and spiritual director of Sakya Losal Choe Dzong and the Rongton Buddhist

Training College in Canberra, Australia. He also guides many affiliated centers across Australia and is the author of several books, including *Lamdre: Dawn of Enlightenment* and *Triple Tantra.*

Marsha Woolf, p. 119, is founder/director of Alternative Resources Unlimited, Inc. II, a nonprofit organization, and of the Tibetan Refugee Health Care Project. She has practiced natural medicine for thirty years, specializing in Chinese and Tibetan methodologies, and is collaborator and clinical director (Tibetan team) of the first FDA-approved clinical trial testing the efficacy of Tibetan medicine in the treatment of metastatic breast cancer. She has traveled regularly to treat patients in Tibetan refugee camps in India. She also coordinates the tours of Dr. Yeshi Dhonden, the eminent Tibetan physician, on his medical rounds in the United States. She is the coauthor of the book *The Rainmaker* and is author of the forthcoming *From Precious Pills to Precious Health.*

Grateful acknowledgment is made to the following for permission to reprint copyrighted material.

Bell Tower for "100 Arms of Compassion" from *Bearing Witness: A Zen Master's Lessons in Making Peace* by Bernie Glassman © 1998 The Zen Community of New York. Reprinted with permission from Bell Tower. Dharma Publishing for "Generosity without Bounds" from *Mother of Knowledge: The Life of Ye-shes Mtsho-rgyo* by Nammkhai sNying-po, translated by Tarthang Tulku and Jane Williams © 1983. Reprinted with permission from Dharma Publishing. George Publications for "Lamp in the Dark" from *George* magazine, December 1997, by John F. Kennedy, Jr. © 1997. Reprinted with permission from George Publications. HarperCollins Publishers for "The Equanimity of All That Lives" from *The Snow Lion's Turquoise Mane: Wisdom Tales from Tibet* by Lama Surya Das © 1992 Jeffrey Miller. Reprinted with permission from HarperCollins. North Atlantic Books for "Transformative Forgiveness" from *Buddhist Women on the Edge: Contemporary Perspectives from the Frontier* by Marianne Dresser. © 1996 Marianne Dresser. Padma Publishing for "Gift of Freedom" for *Finding Freedom: Writings from Death Row.* Jarvis Jay Masters © 1997. Reprinted with permission from Padma Publishing. Parallax Press for "Two Minds One Heart" from *Being Peace* by Thich Nhat Hanh © 1987 Thich Nhat Hanh; "The Bullet That Stops All Wars from *Learning True Love: How I Learned and Practiced Social Change in Vietnam* by Chan Khong © 1993; "Transforming Horror" and "Hugging Meditation" from *Teachings on Love* by Thich Nhat Hanh © 1998. Reprinted with permission from Parallax Press, Berkeley, California. Rigpa Fellowship for "The Highest Prayer" by Sogyal Rinpoche. From a public talk in New York, September 12, 1999 © Rigpa Fellowship; "Pacifying Aggression" recounted by Orgyen Tobgyal Rinpoche, in "Khyenste Ozer: Radiance of Wisdom and Compassion," *International Journal of the Rigpa Fellowship,* August 1990. Reprinted with permission from Rigpa Fellowship. Shambhala Publications for "Simple Care" from *Lovingkindness: The Revolutionary Art of Happiness* by Sharon Salzberg. © 1995 by Sharon Salzberg; "Transforming Anger" from *Start Where You Are: A Guide to Compassionate Living* by Pema Chödrön © 1994; "Taking on the Suffering of Others" from *The Words of My Perfect Teacher* by Patrul Rinpoche © 1994, 1998 by the Padmakara Translation Group. Reprinted with permission of Shambhala Publications. Snow Lion Publications for "Transforming Evil" in *Snow Lion* newsletter, Volume 15, no. 1. Reprinted with permission from Snow Lion Publications. Riverhead Books for "The Supreme Emotion" from *Ethics for the New Millenium,* by The Dalai Lama. © 1999 His Holiness the Dalai Lama. Reprinted with permission from Riverhead Books. Wisdom Publications for "Planting Merit" from *Polishing the Diamond, Enlightening the Mind: Reflections of a Korean Buddhist Master,* by Master Jae Woong © 1999 Korean Buddhist GumGangKyungDokSongHweh Temple; and "All Pervading Kindness" from *The Tantric Distinction: A Buddhist's Reflections on Compassion and Emptiness* © 1999 Jeffrey Hopkins. Reprinted with permission of Wisdom Publications, 199 Elm St. Somerville, MA 02144 U.S.A. www.wisdompubs.org